CW00957387

SICK-NOTE BRITAIN

ADRIAN MASSEY

Sick-Note Britain

How Social Problems Became
Medical Issues

HURST & COMPANY, LONDON

First published in the United Kingdom in 2019 by
C. Hurst & Co. (Publishers) Ltd.,
41 Great Russell Street, London, WC1B 3PL
© Adrian Massey, 2019
All rights reserved.
Printed in the United Kingdom by Bell & Bain Ltd, Glasgow

Distributed in the United States, Canada and Latin America by
Oxford University Press, 198 Madison Avenue, New York, NY 10016,
United States of America.

The right of Adrian Massey to be identified as the author of
this publication is asserted by him in accordance with the
Copyright, Designs and Patents Act, 1988.

A Cataloguing-in-Publication data record for this book
is available from the British Library.

ISBN: 9781787381223

The lyrics of Harvey Danger's 'Flagpole Sitta', from the 1997 album
Where Have All the Merrymakers Gone?, are reproduced with kind
permission of Sony/ATV Music Publishing.

This book is printed using paper from registered sustainable
and managed sources.

www.hurstpublishers.com

CONTENTS

CONTENTS

ACKNOWLEDGEMENTS

Earnest thanks are due to Mike O'Donnell and David Slavin. Both demonstrated the humility and self-deprecating humour of the true subject-matter expert when sharing their many ideas with me, and were instrumental in encouraging me to think and to write. In my early years as a Force medical advisor to the police I was under the tutelage of Mike McCann, and fortunate to be taught the value of common sense, pragmatism and humanity from such a wise mentor.

As the semblance of a book began to emerge, I came to appreciate the importance of ideas, and of intellectual challenge to those ideas, if deeper truths are to be reached. Throughout my association with Hurst they have embodied this ethos. Sickness and disability can be controversial themes, and I am truly grateful for being given the space for free expression and to advance arguments that are long overdue. Lara Weisweiller-Wu in particular merits special mention for her tenacity, rigour and sharp mind, all of which have made this book immeasurably better than my initial manuscript.

My mothers—English and Irish—have been unstinting in their support and encouragement; it has been as a result of the sacrifices made by each that I have been able to enjoy the career and the experiences that I have. Finally, my wife and two boys.

ACKNOWLEDGEMENTS

Writing this book took me away from them more than I wished; I can only hope to reciprocate by being just as supportive in all their endeavours in the years to come.

PREFACE

Sickness rates rose for much of the twentieth century and remain stubbornly high in the twenty-first, despite progressively safer work and better healthcare. It must, then, have complex causes: we should think of it as a crucible where economics, politics, law, morality and medicine collide. Instinctively we focus our efforts on medical interventions as a means of managing sickness, yet these are ineffectual—because the most powerful drivers of sickness are not medical.

This book has one objective: to convince the reader that the principal medical intervention used to manage sickness—the requirement for doctors to certify it—is folly. This is an anachronistic sham that we can ill afford at a time when doctors already lack sufficient time for their core purpose, which is the treatment of ill people. *Sick-Note Britain* is not intentionally political, but it does venture to suggest some logical policy responses. I hope these will stimulate thought about how we would manage in a world where doctors were freed from performing the 'meaningless formality' of certification.[1] Where the reader does not agree with my suggestions, then I hope that this does not detract from the central point that is being made.

In the course of researching this book, the work of Ivan Illich has had a profound influence on my thinking, and is referenced at intervals throughout. Illich was especially concerned about the dehumanising and counterproductive consequences of industrialisation. My personal experiences over the last few years have helped me to develop some insight into these. I grew up in the Midlands in an anonymous commuter town outside of Birmingham. Mine was a typical late-twentieth-century suburban upbringing. I had been adopted at birth but knew nothing of my origins until the advent of my fortieth birthday, when nagging curiosity got the better of me. After some enquiries I learnt that my biological parents were from a rugged, windswept and remote village on the Atlantic coast of County Mayo. In 2014 I was reunited with my biological mother, by then a nurse living in the north of England, with my biological father—a cattle farmer still living in the same village—and with an extended Irish family.

On visiting this remote part of rural Ireland, I began to develop some sense of how very different life would have been, for both good and bad, for most people just a couple of hundred years ago, compared with the experience of city-dwellers today. I have had the unusual experience of being immersed in two very different cultures, feeling rooted to some extent in each, and as a result came to appreciate how much the story of sickness is effectively the story of our industrialisation. I hope the book conveys some sense of this juxtaposition.

I have written from the perspective of the doctor, because I am one and because—by and large—when sickness certification is being performed, it is by doctors. Increasingly other healthcare professionals are also being drawn into the politics of sickness, and many of the comments made here are equally applicable to them. For reasons of clarity and brevity, though, I refer to doctors throughout. As the professionals whose defining skillset is supposed to be diagnosis, doctors attract particular criticism in those chapters that deal with the scourge of medicalisation. There the references are specifically and pointedly directed towards them.

SICKNESS

1

MEASURING THE INDESCRIBABLE

Of the people within our economy who are currently off sick, what proportion do you think are actually capable of work? How could you ever test your hypothesis? Is it possible to measure someone's ability to work in any scientific and objective way if they maintain that they are incapable? Are some impediments to work—loss of a limb, blindness, paralysis—more easily measured than others—pain, fatigue, anxiety?

Where it is obvious that someone is unable to work, do we need doctors to tell us that? Where it isn't obvious, are doctors any better than other people at judging how tired, pained, distressed or anxious someone might be? Might doctors even be worse at doing this than other people? What do we even mean when we talk about ability—or 'fitness'—to work? What kind of work? Do we judge that someone who is capable of work, but who may be harmed or hurt through working, should work anyway? If not, how harmful or hurtful does their work have to be before we excuse them? How can we measure and describe this? These are the questions with which this book is concerned.

In the literal sense, sickness refers to the sensation of being nauseated. Here, though, we are using the sociological sense of the word. When we say that someone is 'off sick', we mean that society has accepted that they are too ill to work and are thereby unable at this point in time to 'produce' as a means of supporting themselves.

The social phenomenon of sickness is as old as *Homo sapiens*— as are the moral conundrums it presents. Because as much as we are motivated by the benevolent urge to help others who are in need, so we are gnawed by the fear that our good nature may make us vulnerable to exploitation. How are we to know who is truly unable to work, despite being motivated to do so, as distinct from those who merely prefer not to? Almost 200 years ago the British philosopher John Stuart Mill reasoned that people were economical beings, in the literal sense of not wanting to expend more effort than necessary. He described man as not just 'a being who desires to possess wealth', but also one 'who is capable of judging the comparative efficacy of means for obtaining that end.'[1] This creature, to whom we can all relate, came to be described by Mill's contemporaries as *Homo economicus*: Economic Man.

It is often lamented that we have a system that increasingly taxes work and subsidises non-work.[i] That is because we do. This movement of money from people who are working to people who are not creates an obvious hazard, a mortal threat to the vigour of societies that do not carefully consider how to constrain it. Because, to the extent that people are motivated by self-interest and desire of material things, they also want an easy life. If it becomes commonplace to believe that one is no worse off, or insubstantially worse off, for not working—because money

---

[i] This is typically attributed to Milton Friedman but is unsourced.

4

is paid regardless—then work is devalued. And since work is ultimately the engine for the prosperity of the nation, so we are all impoverished. The extent of sickness in society clearly needs to be contained, for everyone's sake—not least the sick, whose welfare depends on a healthy economy to support them. What is the scale of the problem currently?

If the patient has a job, then their occupational sickness benefits are paid by their employer. The Confederation of British Industry estimated in 2013 that these costs, and associated costs such as lost output and providing staff cover, exceeded £14 billion per year.[2] For those who are unemployed, the bill for state incapacity benefits (£15 billion in 2016) is footed by the taxpayer.[3] Inevitably, many—in fact, a majority—in our society fear that efforts to regulate sickness are ineffective, and that the system is vulnerable to exploitation by those simply seeking an easier life. The 30th British Social Attitudes survey, in 2013, found that 81 per cent of respondents agreed with the statement that 'large numbers of people these days falsely claim benefits'.[4] There is evidently widespread concern that some of those obtaining benefits are doing so out of laziness or a sense of entitlement and not because they are genuinely unable to work.

To know whether they are justified in feeling this way, we would need to have a means of identifying those who are genuinely unable to work, as distinct from those who are merely disinclined to. But what would we mean by 'genuinely unable'? Sometimes it would be easy for a group of observers—benefit assessors—to reach unanimous agreement that someone was manifestly incapable of work. Their incapacity would be regardless of their doggedness to work, or of any assistance an employer might reasonably give them. This is most obvious in cases of people with severe physical, cognitive or sensory disability, or any combination of the three. There are cases—persistent vegetative state, for example—where anyone would agree that the person is

SICK-NOTE BRITAIN

incapable of work. These are not hard cases. The functional impairment is so obvious that having a medical degree really adds very little to the assessment being undertaken: one of capability, rather than a diagnosis. Nor are such cases particularly representative of the claimant group as a whole. Despite this, media debates about sickness will typically be accompanied by imagery of some of the most vulnerable and disabled people in society.[ii] However, it is not at this extreme that assessment of sickness is especially controversial, but at the margin. And most applications are marginal—ones where a superficially plausible case could be made either way about the person's capability for work—because the majority of claimants have more subtle functional impairment. It is not that they absolutely and demonstrably cannot do a particular thing, but that doing so is an ordeal for them, for instance because it makes them feel more tired, pained, anxious or distressed. It is precisely at this margin that the process of sickness assessment becomes so unreliable, because the barriers to work are more experiential (felt only by the individual), and less observable. There is as yet no scientific, objective means of measuring the extent of phenomena such as pain and tiredness; we can only ask the person to describe their experience for us, within the extent to which their vocabulary—and society's scepticism—allows them to do so.

[ii] Data collected by the Department for Work and Pensions is categorised in such a way that it is of limited use in trying to quantify the proportion of sickness benefit claimants with objective evidence of clinically significant disease. However, the data that is recorded shows that the sum proportion of claimants with disorders of the nervous system, injuries and poisoning, and cardiovascular diseases (which, in sum, we might take as a reasonable proxy for 'disease') has fallen—from about 25% in 1996, to less than 20% by 2007—whilst the proportion of claimants with mental and behavioural health problems, and the inevitable 'other' category, rose from a little

6

MEASURING THE INDESCRIBABLE

There are very few people who would be wholly unable to work if their lives depended on it, but is total inability a humane threshold to use in a civilised society? Do we expect someone with arthritis to crawl into work on their hands and knees if necessary, or someone who is severely depressed to huddle in a ball once they get there? Hopefully not, but if not, where should the bar be set? How are we to define in any meaningful sense how much pain and suffering we would expect somebody to endure before they become worthy of our kindness? Can language convey individual experience with enough precision that one person can truly understand another's suffering; so that they may decide if it is sufficiently severe for that person's sickness to be treated as legitimate?

Ludwig Wittgenstein's observations about the limitations of language were hugely influential on philosophical thought in the twentieth century. He showed how many of the questions that had confounded philosophers since ancient times were simply linguistic riddles: diversionary wastes of time, created by the ambiguities of language. Words that are put together in a grammatically correct sense can still be intellectually nonsensical, as in 'What colour is nine?'. Thus Wittgenstein's wisdom: that when it comes to things that are unknowable and indescribable, 'Whereof one cannot speak, thereof one must be silent.'[iii]

---

over 50% to a little over 60% in the same period. The evidence suggests that the proportion of claimants with what we might term 'non-physical' health problems is high and rising, whilst the proportion with serious and life-threatening disease is low and falling. Researchers from the Institute for Financial Studies have reported on the same trend ('Disability Benefit Receipt and Reform: Reconciling Trends in the United Kingdom').

[iii] The seventh and final proposition, and concluding line of, Wittgenstein's *Tractatus Logico-Philosophicus*.

So it is with attempts to describe in precise terms experiences as subjective and uniquely personal as pain and suffering. Sickness assessment schemes are premised on the assumption that suffering is capable of description and measurement, and then pose a series of nonsense questions about 'fitness for work' to see if applicants measure up. The social division and vitriol that result from these schemes demonstrate how nonsense questions are not just an offense to logic, they can cause real harm. There are some—many—questions we are better off not asking, since they generate confusion rather than clarity.

Even accepting the imprecisions of language, can we rely on the person's own account of how they are feeling? They are neither disinterested in the outcome of our assessment, nor stupid (according to John Stuart Mill, at least). So, how far should we insist on a veterinary approach: recognising only problems that are tangible and capable of being physically measured? And if we could measure human misery, what should be the *Système International* unit of measurement? Perhaps the Job, after the biblical figure whose name is synonymous with suffering: 1.4 Jobs for a kidney stone, 3.4 for an acrimonious divorce, 5.2 for someone feeling exceptionally depressed—that kind of thing?

All attempts at the objective measurement of sickness are nothing of the sort. When someone reports feeling tired, pained, anxious, distressed or otherwise unable to do a particular thing for a particular reason, generally there is no way of proving that they are or aren't exaggerating. In the absence of incontrovertible evidence that the person can do the things they claim not to be able to do—for example, covert surveillance footage—the best anyone can do is to accuse the individual of lying. Yet one of the paradoxes of sickness assessment is that society simply does not allow doctors—the group entrusted to make these assessments on our behalf—to make value judgments of this kind about the individuals they see.

What's more, whatever the extent to which we can get some hazy idea of what the person is experiencing—as distinct from what they report experiencing—it is still a moral judgment on the part of the assessor as to whether the person's suffering is sufficient that they should be excused the obligation to work. What one doctor who reads the *Daily Mail* may consider to be reasonable, their *Guardian*-reading colleague may not.

Different approaches have been taken to the dilemma of how to assess sickness, in different cultures and at different times. None have been wholly satisfactory, though some have been on balance better than others. The situation could be summarised by saying that the material support for sick people has improved enormously as living standards generally have increased, but the efficiency with which sickness is targeted has deteriorated as society has become more complex. This has led to the rancour and cynicism that now typify the debate about social policy when it comes to the sick.

2

TRENCH WARFARE

For the great majority of human history, the politics of sickness have been negotiated in an intensely personal way. During the time when we led a hunter–gatherer existence in caves, through to a life of subsistence agriculture in bucolic hamlets, the transaction between benefactor and beneficiary was direct. Those capable of work would be satisfied that a neighbour was in genuine need through a knowledge of their character that is only acquired by having lived alongside somebody in a small community for a lifetime. That, and according to the evidence of their own eyes and ears. This was a time when incapacity was likely to be caused by the all-too-obvious ravages of disease, pestilence and starvation, rather than the more refined and untestable maladies currently fashionable amongst modern Westerners.

The decision to help was essentially charitable, an unenforced personal decision made according to the person's own means, morality and religious or mystical beliefs. No doubt, this decision was influenced in part by fear of the stigma they would experience were they to fail to do their bit: of being ostracised themselves in their own hour of need. But—very differently from the modern day—help was not given under the coercion of the state, in the guise of the taxman.

Just as it was left to the good conscience of the individual to decide whom they wished to help, they also had choice about the type of support offered. In an age of barter and rudimentary finance, the help would typically have been in kind rather than in cash: food, in a time when calories were scarce; water, when this would have necessitated a gruelling walk to and from the river or well; fuel, when keeping warm required cutting, chopping, carrying and lighting firewood; time, when human company would have been the sole entertainment; or companionship, when ignorance about the causes of disease—or sometimes justifiable fears—might have led many to stay away.

The transaction of sickness became increasingly convoluted with industrialisation. Mass production resulted in our move to anonymous metropolises. First, during the industrial revolution, to work in mines and factories; then, with increasing automation and globalisation, to work in offices. Gradually the administration of relief to the sick became something that was overseen by people with a designated responsibility for this task, mirroring the specialisation of labour that was occurring more widely within society. The process began with the Elizabethan Poor Laws 500 years ago, whereby aid was administered by 'Overseers of the Poor', and continued with the first National Insurance Act of 1911, which designated 'Panel Doctors' and 'Sick Visitors' as the relevant functionaries.[i] With the arrival of the National

---

[i] A later Departmental Committee report into the effectiveness with which sickness benefits were paid under the Act (the Schuster inquiry) contains many contemporaneous accounts of how things were changing. Question 16,498 in the appendix to the report (available at https://archive. org/stream/b21361125_002#page/n47/mode/2up) contains the following passage from a Dr W. Bennett of Liverpool: 'They knew one another, and

Health Service in 1948, family doctors assumed responsibility for certifying sickness on behalf of the new Ministry of National Insurance.

Now, the transaction of sickness is not directly between villagers but facilitated through the tender mercies of a bureaucratic intermediary, be that a corporation (for the employed) or the state (for the unemployed). For the sick worker, support is no longer delivered by their neighbours and workmates but by the human resources team or payroll officer. For the sick without a job, the interaction is with the welfare state in the form of the lumbering behemoth that is the Department for Work and Pensions—the current incarnation of the Ministry of National Insurance.

The DWP is responsible for administering payments relating to work, welfare, pensions and child maintenance. Given that it occupies such a pivotal role in society, it is predictably huge. Its apparatchiks administer a quarter of all government spending (£173 billion in 2015–16, out of a total of £772 billion)[1] and its annual running cost was almost £6.5 billion in the financial year 2015/16.[2] In the same year it spent £15 billion on sickness benefits.[3] For a country estimated to have overspent by £72.2 billion that year, and which accrued total debts of £1.8 trillion by 2017/18, we still feel surprisingly capable of such expenditure.[4]

This intrusion of the state into what was once a matter of individual conscience means that the human aspect of almsgiving has been subverted. Primarily, it has been anonymised: first by the slicing and dicing of taxed income by Her Majesty's Revenue and Customs, and then by the homogenisation of the DWP. Contributions extracted under sufferance from a multitude of

there was a sense of unity amongst them. They realised that their funds were in one another's hands, whereas now, in these societies, you may have people living next door to each other in the same society, but without the faintest idea of the fact.'

anonymous benefactors are puréed and piped out the other end to similarly unidentified recipients. Those on either side of these state colossuses are unknown to one another, with each liable to develop their own *idée fixe* about the other's intentions. For the taxpayer this means that all welfare recipients are imagined as scheming loafers, whilst for claimants (and the groups that represent them) all concerns expressed by taxpayers about levels of expenditure are proof of their fascist credentials. These perceptions endure because the individuals that hold them are denied the human interactions that might moderate their beliefs.

Once the sick would have seen their neighbour pass their window in foul weather and at an ungodly hour to tend to their oxen for them. For their part, their fellow villagers would have witnessed first-hand the patient's pox, consumption and heaving of phlegm and bile. For their modern-day counterparts, the situation is more akin to trench warfare. Each side gets only the merest glimpses of their opposite numbers as they scurry about their day-to-day lives, only too aware of their own personal travails and liable to demonise their invisible fellow citizens. Occasional salvos are lobbed between opposing trenches, which is what passes for political discourse about sickness.

The anonymising effect of the welfare state means there is no longer a no man's land in which to fraternise; no place for a softening of attitudes to occur in the way that villagers from different sides of the street would once have congregated together in church. This was not a conscious, deliberate intention of the welfare state, but rather an inescapable consequence of humanity's trajectory towards social insurance schemes of ever greater complexity. Ironically, to a large extent the charitable ideal has been corrupted by these attempts at enforced, wide-scale charity. In its place we find suspicion, cynicism and animosity.

An asymmetry has developed between the increasing efficiency with which citizens are compelled to pay their tithes in industrialised society—the culmination of which will be our move to a cashless society, whereby Big Brother government has a window into all of an individual's financial transactions[ii]—and the decreasing feedback citizens receive to reassure them that the wealth they have created is being redistributed fairly. As one commentator has put it, in more succinct and neuroscientific terms, 'the phenomena of modern social welfare activate emotional and cognitive systems designed for regulating ancestral small-scale exchange of help'.[5] In other words, the primeval worry that we are being exploited puts us on alert, but the tension is unresolved because we are so remote from the recipients of our help that we are denied the opportunity to satisfy ourselves, through knowledge of their character and direct observations of them, that they are suitably deserving. Instead, and in words bound to send a chill down any spine, we are to trust officialdom to look out for us on our behalf. Yet, in the words of Trotsky, 'Bureaucracy and social harmony are inversely proportional to each other.'[6]

The welfare state is ineffective at bringing together those who sit on opposite sides of the debate regarding sickness benefits: those paying in, and those taking out. This is not for the sake of trying. There have been a number of attempts simultaneously to reassure both taxpayers and claimants that the state, acting as an intermediary, is competent to administer sickness benefits in a way that is fair to everyone. The inevitable failure of these attempts to reconcile competing interest groups, whose agendas are so dia-

---

[ii] Various central banks have already embarked on a programme to remove physical cash from circulation as a means of reducing tax avoidance, typically beginning with higher denomination notes: in 2016 the Reserve Bank of India withdrew ₹1,000 and ₹500 notes; the European Central Bank is discontinuing the €500 note; and South Korea intends to outlaw coins as legal tender by 2020.

metrically opposed, has been painfully apparent in a series of parliamentary reports under the 2010–15 coalition government.

The Work Capability Assessment was launched as part of a welfare reform package in 2010. It was intended as an objective and fair means of assessing eligibility for the new state sickness benefit, the Employment and Support Allowance (ESA). Since it was anticipated that this would be a controversial scheme, Parliament created a legal duty for the work and pensions secretary to provide an annual progress report on the Work Capability Assessment, written by independent reviewers, for the first five years of its operation.[7] Five reports were duly laid before Parliament between 2010 and 2014.

In the first report, concern was expressed that the new system was perceived by recipients as 'impersonal and mechanistic',[8] as though this state-administered exercise in redistributing £8 billion of taxed income could ever be otherwise. Perhaps there was a wistful hope that, in homage to simpler times, the chap from the DWP might occasionally pitch up with a friendly wink, casserole in hand, and a suggestion that—just this once—the paperwork could be overlooked. There was disappointment that, when an application for a benefit was declined, it was not received in a more upbeat manner as a 'positive first step towards work', something that would surely have come as no surprise to John Stuart Mill. This very first report on the Work Capability Assessment, less than a year after its introduction, also contained the revealing observation that 'fairness can mean different things to different people'—a hint of things to come.

By the third year, the report was quoting Machiavelli,[9] an interesting source of inspiration after three years in a ringside seat at the perpetual struggle between those lobbying for claimants and those lobbying for the taxpayer. In 2014 the final report noted that the Work Capability Assessment 'remained controversial', that reforms had taken it 'about as far as it can sensibly go', and that in the future society should consider whether 'health related capability for work is the criterion that [it] wishes to use to determine benefit levels'.[10]

In short, the Work Capability Assessment had singularly failed in its objective to achieve a consensus of opinion that sickness benefits were being fairly administered. To continue the trench warfare metaphor, the reviewers had given up urging each year for one more push—in the manner of a First World War general confident in eventual victory—and instead had succumbed to despair after years of failed attempts to break the stalemate. The final reviewer's valedictory advice was that we should contemplate whether schemes that require sickness to be measured are such a good idea after all—and, of course, they aren't.

As well as blunting our discretion to exercise charity according to our judgment and intuition, and thereby fomenting perpetual grievances within society, 'progress' has debased the currency of human mercy itself. That currency no longer tends to be kindness, food, warmth, or the donation of labour and skills. Although euphemisms are used, with talk of support and benefits, we should be frank and acknowledge that in the modern era the welfare state's demands for consistency and administrative convenience mean that these concepts have a narrow, purely fiscal, meaning. The homogenising effect of the welfare state means that money is now the metric of human charity. An organisation the size of the DWP does not go in for leaving firewood or fresh preserves on people's doorsteps.

This is problematic, as the polite, educated people who are interested in the academic aspects of sickness evidently dislike talking about something as vulgar as money. They devise lengthy and impressive-sounding phrases to describe their theories. These will relate to anything that might conceivably have a bearing on whether or not someone is likely to seek the sick role, save perhaps their star sign. But they don't mention money. The 'biopsychosocial model', currently in vogue, is a case in point. It is hailed as a holistic approach, since it acknowledges that psychological and social factors influence the way people behave just as much as biological factors. For example, workers may decide to call in sick in the mistaken belief that work is likely to be harmful if they are experiencing any level of symptoms, when generally the precise opposite is true: work—with the routine, structure, security and social interaction it offers—is likely to be helpful (see Chapter 3). They may be facing, and understandably prioritising, domestic caring responsibilities for a child or frail relative that conflict with their contractual commitments. As a way of thinking about sickness, the biopsychosocial model is certainly a quantum leap forward from the traditional medical approach, which is based on the naive assumption that illness, sickness and disability are simply consequences of disease. But there is an elephant in the room, or at least an elephant-sized hole.

Money is missing. Incredibly few professionals are so gauche as to point this out during lofty scholarly discussions. Yet imagine constructing a theory looking at the reverse—the reasons why people do work—and failing to mention their wage. The role of money is just as vital as the role of disease to any understanding of sickness in the real world outside of academia, but it is largely neglected for reasons of political correctness and good taste. In the spirit of the awful, polysyllabic, Mary Poppins-inspired names that are given to behavioural theories, we badly need a moralofinanciopsychosociobiological model if we are to include all the factors that influence people's choices about work—and in a more plausible order.

Does this matter? Yes, inasmuch as the gifting of money—rather than the neighbourly benefits-in-kind of yore—further fans the flames of paranoia among those already suspicious about the agenda of anonymous sickness benefit recipients. Money is convertible—into game consoles, satellite television subscriptions, tobacco, alcohol, drugs and holidays as much as to food and heating—in a way that is not true for bread, fuel and blankets. It provides scope for the cynic to attribute any manner of unhealthy motivations to the sick, in a way that traditional acts of practical charity never did. For this reason, periodically a commentator will suggest that modern welfare may have something to learn from the ancestral approach of paying benefits in kind rather than in cash. But their proposition that at least some benefits might be better paid as vouchers—towards food or fuel, for example—will predictably be rejected by others as one that is demeaning to welfare recipients.

The rationale for this objection does not tend to be clearly articulated. There may be some whose understanding of the concept of money is sufficiently slim that they believe some alchemy is involved in giving people cash as opposed to giving them physical items; that somehow the transfer of wealth is less real, and so less insulting or paternalistic, if someone is given money by 'the government' than if they were to come and clear another person's pantry, or make off with their television. But the idea that wealth can be magicked from the ether is patently fatuous. Whether the government passes freshly minted notes to claimants (from its quantitative easing programme), or simply passes on the ones it has received in taxation, when benefits are paid to those not working it must be at the expense of those currently in work. In one case this is achieved through a devaluation of the currency, in the other by a straightforward redistribution of wealth.

Others have a different reason to object to some sort of benefits in kind. They recognise the economic reality that there is no such thing as a free lunch, the argument being that those in receipt of vouchers, for instance, would be more identifiable within society: it would be more obvious who was working and who was claiming. The former would be paying for goods and services with cash, and would have a wider choice of what to buy;

19

the latter would be purchasing a restricted range of 'necessary' items with tokens. Objections to this seems to be based on a tacit assumption that modern welfare systems' obscuring and anonymising the reality of a financial transaction—from the productive to the non-productive—is desirable. It may be anything but that. The idea that being identifiable and thus accountable may be hygienic in the context of welfare payments merits consideration. After all, we normally view the principles of transparency and openness as characteristic of good governance over financial processes in all other areas of public life.

The human act of charity towards the sick was a subtle and imperfect business at the best of times, even before the intervention of the state. Efforts to condense it down to a procedural flow-chart for the expedience of administrators are simplistic; attempts to commoditise it into cold hard cash, funnelled anonymously from taxpayers to claimants, generate an implacable suspicion. A state of permanent hostility prevails.

3

TABLOID TALES

Scrounging is a delightfully expressive word that does not appear in the academic literature about sickness but is firmly in the vernacular. It should have been coined by Dickens but in fact entered usage in the early 1900s, a few decades after his death, as a derivative of the word 'scringe', which meant to glean. Examples of Dickensian antiheroes are everywhere, a staple for tabloid newspapers looking to tap into the sense of moral panic with lurid tales of egregious scroungers and their shameless scrounging. These reliably entertaining content-fillers are the modern-day village stocks.

They include a former 'Mr Wales' who was in receipt of disability benefits whilst participating in bodybuilding contests;[1] an applicant reportedly unable to walk unaided who ran karate classes;[2] somebody who claimed he could walk only 10 yards and who was filmed playing almost 6,500 yards of golf;[3] a man who was supposedly bed-bound most of the time yet was pictured jet-skiing;[4] an agoraphobic applicant who stated that she could not leave her house but was found to be living in India;[5] a man purportedly crippled by arthritis who was filmed energetically jiving at a dance competition;[6] and a town mayor who was filmed marching over a mile during a Remembrance Day service when supposedly incapable of walking more than 10 metres.[7] Clearly we need to be vigilant over our mayors, as another was caught refereeing football matches whilst apparently unable to walk.[8]

It is difficult to keep up. In the course of writing this book, other colourful cases up before the beak have included a lady supposedly unable to walk more than one metre per minute who was pictured snorkelling in the Maldives,[9] and an ex-Paratrooper nicknamed 'Action Man', purportedly unable to walk more than 50 metres, whose achievements included Alpine skiing, winning two triathlons, wing-walking and the ascent of Kilimanjaro.[10] All were no doubt having 'a good day', not only the strapline to adverts for a popular brand of effervescent vitamin drink, but also the hackneyed excuse of benefit cheats caught red-handed. In September 2018 a benefits fraudster 'in constant pain ... [needing] help cooking, washing and dressing himself' was given a suspended nine-month prison sentence after being filmed on a zip wire.[11] In a twist on Juvenal's ancient dilemma,[i] his wife—a member of the DWP's Fraud Investigation Team—was also handed a suspended service, and community service, after the judge did not accept her plea that she had completed her husband's application forms simply because she had the neater handwriting.

Perhaps because of such tales, it is practically impossible for the protagonists of any debate about sickness to refrain from moralising about the issue. There will be those inclined to a more charitable assessment of their fellow man or woman, for whom the suggestion that any benefit fraud occurs at all is a heinous slur on humanity. Writing in *The Guardian* in 2016, the columnist Frances Ryan decried the government's benefit fraud

---

[i] *Quis custodiet ipsos custodes*, 'Who will guard the guards themselves?'

hotline as perpetuating the myth of the 'phantom benefit cheat'.[12] Yet, as the numerous examples above illustrate, the temptation to continue drawing sickness benefit—when an applicant's circumstances have changed, and what was once appropriate is no longer so—is simply too great for some to resist.

Some people are starry-eyed—generally the better-off who, safely insulated from life's grittier realities, are not averse to preaching to the lumpenproletariat that their fear of being cheated out of what little they have is in fact a prejudice, and that they should have greater generosity of spirit. Mill's liberal contemporaries also bridled against his depiction of man as a creature driven by self-interest. When they gave it the moniker of *Homo economicus*, it was with derisory intent. At the other extreme will be those whose cynicism knows no bounds. Foaming keyboard warriors populate the online comments pages of the daily newspapers, struggling to accept that there is anyone in receipt of benefits who does not automatically warrant birching.

The truth is prosaic and somewhere in between. Some degree of shirking seems to be endemic and, within limits, tolerated. According to a 2015 opinion poll of 1,625 people, 19% confessed to having 'thrown a sickie', to use the colloquial, in the preceding twelve-month period.[13] Of the options given to them, 7% of the sample admitted making a report of sickness that was a total fabrication, 7% that they had exaggerated the severity of a minor ailment to avoid work, and 5% that their non-attendance was the result of a hangover. These Ferris Buellers evidently enjoy their days off: a similar poll of 2,000 people about their attitudes to sick days found that, whilst feeling guilty, 63% nevertheless felt they were 'totally worth it'.[14] If you are not one of them, you are obviously missing out. Doubly so if you are having to cover their job. In a third survey from 2006, only 26% of employees 'strongly disapproved' of sickies, although 39% felt 'people shouldn't do this, it's not fair on others'. In other words, 35% had an agnostic or even admiring stance. Seven per cent agreed with the statement 'Good luck to them if they can get away with it'.[15]

Attitudes to the short-term sickness of employed people are about as severe as those towards speeding drivers—literally. The 2011 'National Survey of Speeding Attitudes and Behaviors' by the US Department of Transportation found that 30% of drivers described behaviour on the road identifying them as 'speeders', and that only 67% strongly agreed with the statement that 'Everyone should obey the speed limits because it's the law.'[16] When people kick back a little and have an unofficial day off, or indulge their inner Toad in their motor car, many will tut—but with a wry smile. Few have led such wholly august lives that they are in a position to throw stones.

But attitudes harden when the absence is lengthy and the individual has no job. The vilification of state sickness benefit claimants is more like that of drink-drivers: they are seen less as lovable rogues and more as a social menace.[17] At this point the magnitude of the misdemeanour is such that fewer people can relate to it. These aren't seen as people caught doing 34mph in a 30mph zone, but as the motorcyclist photographed pulling a wheelie at 103mph.[ii] Since the mechanism of benefit is directly through the state, it is more obvious to everyone that ultimately it is they, not a corporation, who are footing the bill, which no doubt is an aggravating factor.

These arguments about where the average person taking sick leave sits on a spectrum of virtue ranging from Mother Theresa

---

[ii] A gentleman by the name of Lukasz Wisniewski can lay rightful claim to this accolade. It was his misfortune to perform the manoeuvre past a camera van in Selby in 2012. The episode is reported in a suitably non-judgmental manner for the enjoyment of other motorcyclists on the 'Motorcycle News' website. It is not reported whether he was pulling a sickie at the time.

to Al Capone are salacious and fun. But they are a major distraction from more considered analysis of the problem of sickness. Stereotyping the characters as either saints or sinners, excluding the possibility of more subtle and complicated explanations, has long acted as an impediment to progress. This is a difficult habit to shake off, as work has long been associated with issues of morality. The Greek aristocracy despised the concept of work as something that was debasing and for slaves; the Protestants took the contrary view of work being integral to the expression of their piety. Both were merely human, metaphysical interpretations of the relative significance (or insignificance) of humankind's battle with the universe's tendency to entropy—what we might consider the most pure, scientific definition of 'work'. For the Greeks, with their clear separation of humankind from the gods, the efforts of the former—and thus the importance of human work—would have appeared trifling. For the Protestants, humans may merely have been the humble tools, but still of God's work itself.

These perspectives represent the extremes of the moral significance that different cultures have attached to work. Neither represents an inherent truth. For the purposes of this book, from here on we can consider that when work is described as important, this is for the worldlier reasons of economy and human health. Also that, generally speaking, maximising participation in work is therefore beneficial for both the individual and society. Work is the engine for getting things done within society and hence—in conjunction with technological improvements that improve our productivity—the key means by which living standards generally are improved, and the most vulnerable cared for. Increasingly work is recognised as key to the public health agenda as the evidence mounts that those in employment live longer, healthier, happier lives than those outside of it.[18]

With these insights, we are finally devising new and more helpful understandings of sickness behaviour, developing theories that better match the evidence. The causes of sickness and the corresponding solutions, in a practical rather than a puritanical sense, are becoming clearer.

Despite what the media would have you believe, normally when someone is sick from work it is not a calculated or deliberate act on their part. Except for those employed in the public sector (who typically receive full pay for the first 6 months of their absence), or those working in the private sector with unusually generous sick pay (usually for large corporates), long-term absence is a meagre life.[iii] Generally it is not the permanent holiday that people who have never endured lengthy periods of purposelessness might imagine. Instead sickness is frequently the result of the unhelpful actions—or failure to act—of other people. If we must moralise about sickness then it is important to recognise that often the blame needs to be shared around rather than directed at the most obvious target. We need to learn to hate the game, not the player.

Once, we may have thought solely in terms of the deserving and the undeserving sick; the genuine and the malingerers. I do not claim that fraudsters do not exist—as we have seen from the press cuttings, and contrary to what Frances Ryan would have you believe, they undeniably do—but this is a fairly binary way of thinking and in most cases it won't help us to properly under-

---

[iii] At the time of writing in October 2018, even the highest level of award under the Employment and Support Allowance award (for those in the Support Group, with the Enhanced and Severe Disability premiums) is £262.90 per week. Those who think that sickness benefit claimants are an easy target point out, fairly in my view, that if there is anger about the nation's perilous finances it might be better directed at the financial sector. The National Audit Office calculated that the cost of the bailout after the 2008 crisis amounted to £850 billion; the annual sickness benefit bill is 0.0018% of that figure.

stand what is going on. Instead it is more helpful to think in terms of the avoidably and unavoidably sick. These terms do not carry the same moralistic connotations; if there is blame it is not necessarily attached to the individual, though it may be. Framing things this way allows a more dispassionate consideration of the problem, which in turn leads to more rational solutions. When a team has conceded a goal, the goalkeeper is an easy target; but the calamity may have begun much further up the field.

It is a fact of life that in any population there will be a minority of people with health problems sufficiently disabling that no-one would reasonably expect them to work. These are the unavoidably sick, or the deserving sick as the moralisers might prefer. They are a group that will always exist and will always need our help. Unfortunately, some rehabilitation experts have difficulty leaving them alone. This is an unfortunate side-effect of their desire to right past wrongs. In a former age, healthcare professionals had ridiculously high anxiety about the mortal peril that returning to work and wielding a pen might pose, and they advised people against it wherever possible; many still do. Like a stopped clock, their advice would occasionally have been correct, even if it was mindlessly given. There is a danger that, now they have been enlightened about the health-giving properties of work—and these are substantial—they get carried away. Some today have transitioned from indiscriminately telling everyone that they shouldn't work to telling everyone that they should.

The hope and inspiration for severely disabled people, derived from examples such as Douglas Bader and Stephen Hawking, can be taken too far. Bader and Hawking were extraordinary men, but we cannot all be extraordinary. Also, their achievements were at their own instigation; they were their own taskmasters. No-one would have harangued Bader as a failure had he never flown again, or Hawking were he to have ceased theorising. The situation is very different when it is a third party, judging on behalf of the person's employer or the DWP, what someone 'should' be capable of doing. If it were a matter of life or death nearly everyone could work but, as we have established, in a civilised society this should not be the test. Self-evidently the more appropriate test is whether we might reasonably expect the person to work. This is one reason why attempts at supposedly objective assessments of sickness are nothing of the kind. Logically, when the apparently simple concept of fitness for work is deconstructed, it becomes clear that the assessor's answer depends as much on their prejudices as on their skills in determining the level of disability. What puritans might consider 'reasonable', liberals may not, and vice versa.

A minority of profoundly ill people are the exception to the rule that sick people should try to work. The rehabilitation zealots need to be careful: proselytising to people trapped in the most unfortunate circumstances, preaching that work can help to set them free, will result in unfavourable comparisons.[iv] The unavoidably sick rightly belong on benefit schemes and deserve to be left unmolested. However, it is a mistake to think that that help must necessarily be delivered in the form of sickness benefits: a co-ordinated system of disability benefits and a universal out-of-work benefit would be a much better solution (see Chapter 21).

If we accept that keeping people in work despite their illnesses is a team effort, and that strikers, midfielders and defenders can ruin our chances just as much as goalkeepers, then the idea that someone might be avoidably sick but nevertheless deserving of our help does not seem so strange. They may have fallen out of

---

[iv] The mantra of modern-day vocational rehabilitation is that 'work is good for you' (now revised to 'good work is good for you'). Sceptics have observed that this is uncomfortably close to the phrase 'work makes you free', which, in its German form (*Arbeit macht frei*), was emblazoned on the gates to Auschwitz and various other concentration camps.

work because, in their time of need, they were let down by the rest of the team. This is a hugely important group, because they represent the majority of people who are sick and, crucially, because something can be done about their predicament. We can train the other team members—their managers, the healthcare professionals who treat them, even their families—to be less Kidderminster Harriers and more Manchester United, with all apologies to Kidderminster. In other words, improving the support that they receive will enable them to rejoin the workplace—which is where this group of people belong.

Finally, there are those who are avoidably sick, but as a result of a deliberate fraud; the pantomime villain benefit scroungers so beloved of the red-tops. They attract a disproportionate amount of attention whilst constituting, in reality, a fairly small part of the problem of avoidable sickness. The overwhelming majority of sickness benefits are now paid in the form of the Employment and Support Allowance (£14.5 billion out of a total of £15 billion spent on sickness benefits).[19] The DWP's estimate is that 1.7 per cent of ESA payments in 2015/2016—£250 million—were fraudulent, based on the findings of its Fraud Investigation team.[20] Admittedly these are difficult figures to trust; a further £80 million is said to leach from the system as a result of 'genuine' error on the part of claimants in reporting their circumstances to the DWP, and differentiating the two will not always be straightforward.

Even if the DWP's is a substantial underestimate of the total scale of sickness benefit fraud, the overall sum is still likely to remain small in relative terms. Plus, there are unexpected fringe benefits to the fraudsters' activities. Covert surveillance of their capers is sometimes shared with media outlets by the government.[21] The gentle amusement offered by watching these DWP-sponsored editions of *You've Been Framed* seems to atone somewhat for the crime, a return on the taxpayer's involuntary investment in the production costs. The DWP is potentially missing a trick by distributing the footage free of charge. With savvy copyrighting, they could probably break even on the sum that has been defrauded. Even so, aside from any extent to which their antics may lift our spirits, such people unquestionably belong in court.

4

A TWO-WAY STREET

So far we have only considered the responsibilities of the well towards the sick. Already it is apparent that there are difficult questions of ethics and fairness, which the clunky mechanics of the welfare state—or the Human Resources department of MegaCorp®—address more crudely than when it was a matter of human mercy between individuals who knew one another personally. But the definition of sickness provided in Chapter 1 was incomplete; the sociological phenomenon of sickness has a second aspect we should also consider. It is a two-way street, since, although it feels increasingly uncomfortable to mention it, there are the responsibilities of the sick towards the well as much as those of the well towards the sick.

Those familiar with the history of the welfare state, and the principles held dear by its architects, have decried how today's system has morphed into a grotesque caricature of what was intended. The system had its origins in Sir William Beveridge's wartime report *Social Insurance and Allied Services* (the Beveridge Report).[1] This was the blueprint for a better postwar society. Its publication on 1 December 1942 was timely: just weeks after the

El Alamein campaign, a turning point in the war when confidence in ultimate victory over the Axis powers became established and the nation could begin to dare contemplating the postwar world. The welfare state as we understand it was later realised by the 1945–51 government of Clement Attlee, which implemented various Acts, expanding the existing National Insurance scheme and creating the National Health Service.[i]

Beveridge's report was a means of defining a utopian future in a sufficiently tangible way to help sustain the populace during the remaining years of fighting. It was an echo of Lloyd George's promise to create a 'land fit for heroes' at the end of the First World War. Beveridge identified the 'five giant evils' that had bedevilled interwar society—squalor, ignorance, want, idleness and disease—and proposed credible ways in which, by working together, postwar society could address them. The belief that the social unification achieved by the war effort would eventually lead to something uniquely good helped to justify the tragedy and sacrifice again being made by all social classes.

The guiding principles of the Beveridge Report are worth mentioning. One was that social security should be achieved 'by cooperation between the state and the individual'.[2] Another was that the level of security provided should be a minimum, so as not to stifle incentive: 'it should leave room and encouragement for voluntary action by each individual to provide more than that minimum for himself and his family.'[3] In the contemporary narrative Beveridge has been romanticised as an avuncular figure, so

---

[i] Namely, the Family Allowances Act 1945, National Insurance (Industrial Injuries) Act 1946, National Insurance Act 1946, National Health Service Act 1946, Pensions (Increase) Act 1947, Landlord and Tenant (Rent Control) Act 1949, National Insurance (Industrial Injuries) Act 1948 and National Insurance Act 1949.

it jars a little to read his words from his wilder days, when he was by all accounts an avid eugenicist. He wrote chillingly in 1906— admittedly at the tender age of twenty-seven—that

> Those men who through general defects are unable to fill such a 'whole' place in industry, are to be recognised as 'unemployable.' They must become the acknowledged dependents of the state ... but with the complete and permanent loss of all citizen rights—including not only the franchise but civil freedom and fatherhood.[4]

Presumably these attitudes had mellowed by the time he wrote his eponymous report at the age of sixty-three. But even then, although a Liberal, he was emphatically not of the bleeding-heart variety. At the core of the Beveridge Report was the theme of people having mutual responsibilities to one another. He had carried with him his profound convictions about the moral virtue of industry. It is significant that he identified idleness as a great evil in its own right.

Beveridge foresaw a danger that those in receipt of benefits could become accustomed to their new way of life. He proposed that those who had been on long-term benefits 'should be required as a condition of continued benefit to attend a work or training centre, such attendance being designed both as a means of preventing habitation to idleness and as a means of improving capacity for earning.' It was clarified that in part this was a 'way of unmasking the relatively few persons ... who have perhaps some concealed means of earning which they are combining with an appearance of unemployment'.[5] This idea was revived a full sixty-six years and two days later by Paul Gregg, a professor of economic and social policy. On 3 December 2008, in response to a request from the secretary of state for work and pensions, he published a review advocating that very similar conditionality should apply to benefit claimants—in the form of the now-infamous Work Capability Assessment.[6]

Beveridge was an austere man—apparently prone to a daily 6am cold morning bath[7]—who detested idleness, believed in the necessity of cooperation between citizen and state, and who understood that the work ethic is not evenly distributed amongst our brethren. He was a man in tune with the prevailing morality of his times, as evidenced by the eagerness with which the public lapped up his report. Within fifteen months of publication, over 600,000 copies had been sold.[8] It was translated into German and airdropped over the Reich in a propaganda campaign. At the end of the war a Nazi analysis of the text was reportedly found in Hitler's bunker, pronouncing it 'superior to the current German social insurance in almost all points'.[9]

At the time of Beveridge's death in 1963, the welfare state was only seventeen years old. Many have speculated how he might react on seeing his creation now it is a septuagenarian. One biographer suggested that 'He'd be quite horrified by the current welfare state. His system was designed to support economic activity to the fullest extent. He'd think that was not the case today.'[10] The money given to sick people comes largely without strings attached. Largely, but not entirely: there is the minimum expectation that in return the person should do all they can to try and get better and back to work as quickly as possible. The self-evident morality of this scarcely requires further comment. Those who fall on hard times and who end up sofa-surfing at the houses of kind-hearted friends should not get too accustomed to the hospitality of their hosts. Note, the responsibility on the sick is not to return to work—because for some that will not be possible despite any amount of effort—but at least to try.

Without trying, who is to know what is possible, except in the small minority of cases where the odds are manifestly unbeatable? And, as exceptional people such as Douglas Bader illustrate, situations that are truly futile may be rarer than we presume.[ii] We should be wary of underestimating the potential tenacity of human will. The belief that people are automatically disabled by the challenges their malfunctioning bodies and minds might pose for them is a dehumanising one, traducing them to the status of robots. This is one of the criticisms traditionally levelled at the travesty that is the medical model of disability—there are plenty of others.

The sentiment that there is a vice versa, that the sick have a duty to the productive as well as the other way around, is not altogether unreasonable, you might think. Especially if you go to work and pay taxes, and therefore have some skin in the game. But in an age of moral relativism, this is ground where angels— and academics with an interest in the reform of sickness policy— fear to tread. They avoid the 'F' word (fairness) as much as the 'M' one. The quid pro quo of sickness, that there is an onus on the individual to try and alleviate their own plight whilst drawing benefit, tends to be overlooked. Attempts at introducing the principle into sickness benefit schemes are controversial.

One high-profile victim has been Dame Carol Black, a rheumatologist who had already produced two reports for government in 2008 and 2011 with suggestions for policy reforms that would help to reduce sickness, for the benefit of the public health and the economic prospects of the UK.[11] Both had generally been well received. She was, to use the tabloidese, a sickness tsar. Her star fell when in 2015 she agreed to a government request to

---

[ii] In fact, Bader's story shows how adversity can sometimes even provide unanticipated advantages. It was because of his prosthetic legs—having lost both legs in an aircraft crash in 1931—that he was able to survive the shooting down of his Spitfire over Le Touquet in 1941. One foot had become trapped beneath a pedal and he was only able to bail because he could detach his leg. Physiologists have also pointed out that he had a

write a report into whether sickness benefit claimants who were obese or had drug and alcohol addiction should have their payments stopped. A press release from the government lamented the concern 'that not enough is being done to ensure people get help for [these] long-term, potentially treatable issues', before a discreet mention that the review would 'consider the case for linking benefit entitlements to accepting appropriate treatment or support'.[12] *The Sun* reported the news less diplomatically, in an article titled 'Fat's all folks', and predicted that the prime minister would be telling 'fatties, drug addicts and boozers to shape up or risk losing handouts of around £100 a week.'[13]

Agreeing to chair the inquiry may have endeared Black to *Sun* readers and members of the Taxpayers' Alliance, or indeed anyone who dislikes paying taxes, under sufferance, to subsidise other people's vices. But it was never going to win her many friends among the intelligentsia. Predictably this foray into the morality of sickness attracted strong criticism. The president of the Royal College of Psychiatrists, Sir Simon Wessely, coauthored an article in *The Guardian* that described the proposal to remove benefits from people who drink, inject drugs or consume more calories than they expend as 'probably illegal, unethical, impractical and [not likely to] save money.'[14] Those against the government's suggestion to even investigate the proposal could not be accused of sitting on the fence.

---

combat advantage because, when manoeuvring violently, he could sustain greater G-forces than his adversaries without losing consciousness. They blacked out sooner because, as blood pooled in their legs, it was drained from their brains. We tend to overlook how differences that can be disabling can also be advantageous. There are more mundane examples than that of a legendary fighter ace; for example, the high prevalence of obsessive–compulsive disorder amongst accountants, which has been observed anecdotally by many occupational physicians.

In a couple of radio interviews during 2016, Black hinted towards some regrets about accepting this poisoned chalice from then-Prime Minister David Cameron.[15] Her first couple of reports had been sufficiently ivory tower that they had not had to confront any glaring issues of morality. They were very effective in driving sensible and long-overdue reform to the procedural aspects of welfare policy. In contrast, this first skirmish with questions of fairness was enough for the balloon to go up. The report was scheduled for publication in late 2015 and in fact materialised a year behind schedule,[16] probably after a few long dark nights of the soul and—notably—a few months after David Cameron, the instigator of the affair, had resigned as prime minister. There was the suggestion that all claimants, not just those misusing drugs and alcohol, 'attend an early, structured discussion with an appropriate healthcare professional about the barriers to a return to work'.[17] Certainly not the interview without coffee, targeted specifically to those whose moral virtue was in question, that the puritans had been hoping for.

Unsurprisingly, in such a politicised and febrile atmosphere, the central question—about sanctioning benefits for people deemed not to be doing all they could to become capable of work—was fudged. The report stated that there was 'doubt [whether such sanction] should be the first response to the evident problems for the cohorts under discussion', a classic exercise in British understatement and obfuscation. It was left deliberately unclear whether, if not the first response, sanctioning might ever be appropriate as the second, third or nth response. The request from government had simply been a call for evidence. It asked for a report to investigate the merits of the proposal, and appointed a respected academic with a track record of providing constructive and evidence-based recommendations to a succession of Labour, coalition and Conservative governments. That there was outrage from the off shows how sensitive this subject—judging the moral virtue of sickness benefit recipients—has become.

I am not suggesting that withdrawing benefits from the obese or from addicts is necessarily a good or bad idea. Maybe there are some very good practical reasons for maintaining their benefits even if the morality may be questionable; it's clear there are political ones. The point is this: when special interest groups lobby that taxpayers should be compelled to support their agendas, this goes largely unchallenged, but the same is not true in reverse. The mere suggestion that society might be entitled to expectations of how sick people should behave, as much as sick people might have expectations about the regularity of their cheques, was sufficient to ignite the debate.

This affair is not at all surprising in a culture that struggles to acknowledge basic principles of fairness in the confusion generated by an obsession with victimhood and of people being 'shamed'.[iii] Morally justifiable attempts to incorporate into social policy the principle that sick people also have responsibilities have been disparaged as 'sick shaming'. The furore over the Black request is a political manifestation of this phenomenon. It plays

---

[iii] I suspected that the 'shaming' fad was of relevantly recent origins, and Google Trends analytic data suggests as much. There was a 50-fold increase in the word being mentioned in internet searches in the first week of September 2012–for reasons I have not been able to fathom—and it has remained a much more frequent search term since then. The Google data suggests that common searches using the term include cat shaming, passenger shaming, pet shaming, dog shaming, fat shaming, fit shaming, skinny shaming, people shaming, Facebook shaming, public shaming, body shaming and slut shaming. I would suggest that, as a digital record for posterity of quite how self-absorbed and infantile a culture can become, and how rapidly, the shaming phenomenon takes some beating: but that may attract allegations of shaming shaming.

out in a more commonplace way in consultation rooms up and down the country, when doctors, asked to provide a sick-note, ponder the wisdom of being honest. After all, some patients consider it a grievous offence to be reminded of their responsibility to try, as far as they're able, to get better enough to return to work. Sometimes the shock is so great that they feel it may even have delayed their recovery, which poses an interesting logical conundrum as to how they are ever meant to be encouraged back into work.

The potential for such a shock may be convenient in the context of a Work Capability Assessment organised by the Department for Work and Pensions, thanks to an extraordinary piece of statute—namely, Regulation 35(2)(b) of the Employment and Support Allowance Regulations (2008). This enshrines in law the principle that if an applicant for the sickness benefit ESA is considered capable of engaging in 'work-related activity', but that being advised of this fact might cause them significant psychological harm, they should be under no obligation to actually prepare for work.[18] The reader who remains innocent about the finer points of state sickness benefit schemes may wish to reread this paragraph.

There is no doubt that a proportion of applicants to sickness benefit schemes are extremely vulnerable, hence the concern that being fed through the sausage machine that is the DWP might be a bruising and sometimes fatal experience.[19/20] The press has reported numerous cases of suicide, allegedly related to the stress of these encounters with automatons and computers that say no.[21/22/23/24] They represent a small proportion of the total number of applicants, but are all nevertheless tragic. That said, it takes a special kind of thinking, in a society that insists on the 'genuineness' of sickness being tested but where no public official wishes to carry the can when things go wrong, to arrive at the contrived solution adopted in Regulation 35(2)(b).

The logical lesson to draw from these tragedies is that the lumbering bureaucracy of the state can never hope to replicate the kindly, personal, human charitable transactions of years gone by. Any attempt at scaling up a process as subtle and complex as testing claims to sickness is going to be imperfect. The honest approach would be for our executive to level with the electorate: there will always be a human cost to any scheme that involves gatekeeping of sickness benefits, and this cost can only be avoided entirely by abandoning the principle that claimants should be put through their paces. In other words, it is inevitable, unless we revisit the whole idea of targeting benefits according to our judgement of whether or not people are 'genuinely' sick.

This was the conclusion of the valedictory independent review of the Work Capability Assessment. This final reviewer hinted heavily that schemes requiring sickness to be objectively assessed are unworkable and should simply be abandoned on principle, rather than being tinkered with in an interminable series of iterative reforms. That, however, wasn't the policy response that was adopted in response to concerns that the Work Capability Assessment may pose a mortal risk to the most pitiable claimants. Instead, in a society that wants to have its cake and eat it—that wants to interrogate aspiring scroungers and yet also to spare those who may be desperate—we have the legal carbuncle that is Regulation 35(2)(b). Efforts are ongoing to design a system that can both assess 700,000 cases per year,[25] and also retain the necessary sensitivity to detect the needles in the haystack: the quietly desperate people amid the clamour of noisy and entitled ones.

In 2014 the independent review providing an annual commentary on the 'workings' of the Work Capability Assessment noted, with apparent surprise, that Regulation 35(2)(b) was now the route by which 38 per cent of claimants accepted onto the higher tier of ESA were able to access benefit.[26] In other words, of those claiming this benefit, which is intended for people so disabled that they should not have to contemplate work or work-related activity, 38 per cent were actually considered capable of it, but were not advised of this for fear of the psychological harm the news might cause: for example, in situations where a claimant has indicated that they intend to kill themselves if declined benefit.

Such a scenario was entirely predictable. It was envisaged by John Stuart Mill, and by the psychiatrist Andrew Malleson, who has written about the leverage that those who threaten suicide can have over others in a blame-shifting culture. He observed in 1973 that 'suicide threats are a popular and effective way of exploiting the benefits of the welfare state',[27] and thirty-five years later Regulation 35(2)(b) legitimised the process. It is a manifestation of the cognitive dissonance that arises when society requires claims of sickness to be robustly tested on the one hand whilst, on the other, it is exquisitely sensitive to the prospect of causing any harm to vulnerable people and wishes to avoid doing so at all costs. It is impossible to achieve both. Whilst some applicants threatening suicide do so out of genuine desperation, for others it is a calculated manipulation. Yet there is no means of confidently telling them apart and no-one is prepared to be blamed for getting it wrong.[iv]

The Regulation is an unsatisfactory fudge. If we must 'test' sick people then we are better off with it than without it, but why must we test them at all? Perhaps the better solution would be to devise social policy that didn't require vulnerable people to be interrogated in this way in the first place.

[iv] In May 2011 *The Guardian* reported that the DWP had recently circulated a memorandum to its staff stating: 'Some customers may say they intend to self-harm or kill themselves as a threat or a tactic to "persuade", others will mean it. It is very hard to distinguish between the two ... For this reason, all declarations must be taken seriously.' John Domokos, *The Guardian* (8 May 2011). 'Jobcentre staff "sent guidelines on how to deal with claimants' suicide threats"'.

CERTIFICATION

5

DOCTOR PRIESTS

As the welfare state became established the citizenry lost—inevitably—much control over how their income was redistributed. What once was theirs to give or withhold as they saw fit, the state now administers on their behalf. Nowadays the amount of wealth redistributed by the state outstrips the amount given at the discretion of the individual, in charitable donations, by a factor of seventeen.[1]

The compensation for this loss of autonomy has been twofold. First, the establishment of a parliamentary democracy means that individuals decide who is sent to the executive to make the laws under which they will live. The electorate has a say in what proportion of the national wealth should be diverted to welfare, and how it should be distributed–albeit in a much less direct and specific way than when citizens were the master or mistress of their own purse. Secondly, bureaucratic instruments have been devised to govern the administration of welfare and to reassure the populace that, even if they aren't able personally to ensure that their money is being spent wisely, the state will assume this fiduciary responsibility on their behalf. In other words, the suggestion that doctors could be used to ensure that only the deserving sick can access sickness benefits was a sop to the taxpayer, to compensate them for the loss of control over how their own money is spent.

Asking doctors to certify things they cannot possibly know—as distinct from actual doctoring, which is the care and treatment of ill people—is a hallmark of self-styled progressive bureaucracies. In 1766 the Hapsburg Empress Maria Theresa decreed that her court physician should certify the fitness of her subjects to undergo torture, to ensure reliable testimony.[i/2] In these more civilised times, disgruntled applicants to state sickness benefit schemes—trudging their way to a different kind of inquisition, the Work Capability Assessment at the behest of the DWP—might think themselves lucky. Whatever bureaucratic horrors and mental anguish they may be about to face, it will not be physical torture.

In what we smugly think of as a more enlightened age, we scoff at the farcicality of the empress' request. It is so surreal it might have been a Monty Python skit. But the truth is that the policy proposals made within our modern bureaucracies are no less eccentric. In 2017 the German Green Party made the thought-provoking suggestion that doctors might have a role in certifying whether a patient was eligible for state-subsidised access to the services of a prostitute. This would be according to

---

[i] Since the Middle Ages torture had been used to establish the truth in witchcraft trials, and whilst the empress was a reformer she was opposed to its outright abolition. Similarly her physician, Gerard van Swieten, whilst regarded as an Enlightenment figure who understood that many allegations, and behaviours that provoked them, were the product of mental illness, maintained that in some cases there was the possibility of demonic possession. Thus the 1766 edict, by which the two sought to regulate rather than abolish torture.

whether or not 'they are unable to achieve sexual satisfaction in other ways, as well as to prove they are not able to pay sex workers on their own'.[3] The doctor is presumably expected to make a rather unseemly assessment of the patient's upper limb function, as well as somehow having a peculiarly intimate knowledge of their financial circumstances.

This mission creep, whereby bureaucracies consider the remit of the doctor to include assessing the financial as well as biological vicissitudes of their patients, has been evident elsewhere on the Continent too. In 2018 a Belgian doctor who provided a note to excuse a patient on medical grounds from her €70-per-month gym contract—because he did not believe she had sufficient funds and felt under a duty to act 'out of social concern'—was cleared of malpractice by his regulator, Belgium's Order of Physicians. Naturally, the director of Belgium's professional association of gyms had a different view, suggesting that doctors were under a duty to assess someone's health, rather than the wisdom of their financial decisions, and pondering whether they might now adjudicate patients' disputes with their energy or internet suppliers too. Consumer groups in Belgium have long been complaining about expensive and rigid gym membership contracts; but it is difficult to see that the solution has anything to do with doctors.[4]

The phenomenon of GANFYD—Get A Note From Your Doctor—is one of the many miseries inflicted on the modern-day GP that take them away from their actual role of treating patients for medical problems. It can be schools who mistrust parents to make sensible decisions as to whether their own children are well enough to do PE; organisers of extreme sports events seeking assurance that participants looking for an adrenaline rush will not inconveniently drop dead when they get it; airlines seeking confirmation that passengers have a medical need to travel with 'emotional support animals' such as ducks and peacocks;[5] or building firms requiring construction workers to demonstrate a medical need for growing a beard because of the difficulties this can cause when wearing a dust mask.[6/ii]

Or indeed, employers seeking affirmation that when someone says they do not feel well enough to go to work, that is actually how they are feeling. A sick certificate, in the great scheme of things, is no more or less absurd than any of the other things doctors are asked to attest to. GANFYD is the ruse by which organisations intend to avoid risk, cost, inconvenience or controversy by treating the individual as a child and foisting responsibility for their decisions onto a hapless doctor instead. Yet, by putting up their brass plaque, the GP has only advertised their competence in managing health problems in a primary care setting. They have never professed the ability to understand a child better than its own parent, to mind-read, or to have any reliable means of knowing how their gelatinous patient—whose exertion is normally limited to lifting a television remote—will react to being hurled off a viaduct on a bungee cord.

Clearly there is some part of the human psyche, manifest in the behaviour of bureaucracies, that yearns to outsource difficult and potentially unpopular decisions. Who should be tortured, for instance; who should have state-subsidised access to the oldest profession, be allowed to grow a beard, fly with a duck, leap from a bridge attached to an elastic cord, or be signed off sick. If people were to make their own judgements about controversial matters, they would have to assume responsibility for the decision. Yet, in the words of Giosuè Borsi, 'The great thought, the great concern, the great anxiety of men is to restrict, as much as

---

ii One wag contributing to an online doctors' forum about the proposal suggested 'chronic weakchinitis' as an explanation the employer might be prepared to accept.

possible, the limits of their own responsibility.' That is why committees breed sub-committees, steering groups, and expert panels at an exponential rate. It is also why the absurd game of GANFYD remains so popular. For its instigators, it is critical that there must be someone else to whom difficult decisions can be delegated; the existence of evidence that they are especially good at making them is a bonus rather than a prerequisite. The key thing is that there is someone else to blame. In the words of Canadian philosopher Marshall McLuhan, 'the medium is the message':[7] it is not the sense of what is being said that matters, but the fact that it is contained in a note from a doctor.

This is an explanation presented by cynics for the existence of organised religion. Whether that is fair is a matter for theologians, but as a way of understanding social policy and its excessive confidence in experts it has much to commend it. We don't question, because it is more convenient to believe. But why are doctors the group so often in the crosshairs of visionaries such as the German Greens? It is an intriguing question: why are they the ones so regularly invoked as the panacea to awkward, fatuous or risky social dilemmas?

The answers lie in our cultural heritage, and relate to the evolving role of the medicine man in human society. It is not difficult to imagine that the human disposition towards mysticism would lead communities in the prescientific era to believe a select few people had extraordinary abilities of intuition. These might have included the ability to predict or influence the weather, or to communicate with dead ancestors in the spectral realm. In a culture inclined to believe this, how much more tempting to suppose that they would summon that power in the interests of our personal survival, should we fall ill. It would have been an especially attractive and comforting thought. Belief in supernatural power would have been effectively synonymous with belief in the ability to heal, and projected onto the same special group: their shamans or witch doctors. Culturally the concepts of treating disease on the one hand and having some paranormal ability on the other became blended a long time ago.

The modern medical doctor has dispensed with witchcraft, but the presumption that they possess extraordinary perceptual abilities still lingers to a surprising extent. Only the accoutrements of our superstition have changed. Whereas once the wise men were distinguished by their skin paint, drum and feathers, our village elders possess the garb and equipment of the Western physician: the stethoscope, and sphygmomanometer. Few in Western society today would be able to attribute the power of doctors to any magical phenomena with a straight face, mysticism having been expunged from our culture since the Enlightenment onwards. Instead our healers are assumed to derive their intuition from the lengthy medical training that separates them from the layperson. This is an explanation more in keeping with the zeitgeist of a rational age and, since most people have no sense of what the medical apprenticeship entails, an appropriate sense of secrecy and mystery is maintained.

This faith in the capability of doctors is a comforting belief system, reinforced for each generation as a result of the imprinting of trips to the doctor on small children. When a child is deemed in need of a visit to The Doctor the adults will generally discuss the pending encounter in respectful and even reverential terms. This establishes the family doctor's status as an authoritative figure in the adults' lives and, by extension, even more so in the life of the child. One must brush one's teeth and put on clean underwear prior to the consultation for fear of all manner of sordid conclusions The Doctor will otherwise be able to deduce about you. This power play extends into adulthood. The Doctor will see you now; it is Doctor's Orders; you are Under the Doctor.

DOCTOR PRIESTS

Polling consistently reveals that trust in doctors remains substantially higher than for most other professions.[iii] In large part this is an earnt trust, but it would be conceited to assume that social conditioning has not had some hand in this. No doubt many tribes think similarly highly of their healers. This concept of the doctor as a kind of priest, delegated to perform certain social functions by the community on the basis of their having powers that others lack, crops up commonly in anthropology.[8] Ivan Illich used copious religious metaphor in his seminal book *Limits to Medicine* with references to doctors as priests, treatment acts as rituals, and hospitals as cathedrals to the sick.[9] The medicine man is not just an antediluvian concept; he (and it would invariably have been a he back then) followed us from our life in the tribe to our life in the metropolis.

The analogy is not so contrived. Hearing the patient's story is akin to taking their confession. The exchange takes place in the privacy of the clinic room, equivalent to the confessional. Physical examination constitutes the laying on of hands. The act of validation, providing the sick-note or sick certificate, is the bureaucratic equivalent of anointment: absolving the sick from their sin of sloth. Being declined entry to the ranks of the sick is, if accepted with good grace, repentance—a different route to absolution. No record of the encounter is kept by the priest, and what notes are scrawled by the doctor can never be deciphered again by anyone anyway.

[iii] The Ipsos MORI Veracity Index has tracked data about public trust in the professions for some years. Traditionally doctors have always topped the poll; in 2015, 89% of those canvassed expressed confidence in doctors to tell the truth, compared with 49% for NHS managers, 25% for estate agents and 21% for politicians. Notably in 2016 nurses were included in the poll for the first time and immediately displaced doctors from the top spot (93% versus 91%).

51

The myth of doctors having some kind of mystical and priestly intuition, then, remains alive and well even in the age of reason. As we have seen, it has been invoked in relation to matters as diverse as suitability for torture and onanistic capability and, more mundanely, sickness certification. With industrialisation and the emergence of the welfare state, individuals have had less and less scope to support their sick neighbours according to their discretion, and the process has become increasingly remote and anonymous. In compensation for this loss of control, the citizenry needed to be persuaded that sickness was being policed on its behalf by a suitably wise and perceptive professional class. Doctors, with all this cultural baggage, fitted the bill perfectly.

6

SICK-NOTES

The charade of having to traipse down to your GP surgery in order to convince them that you are correct in saying that you feel to ill too work—when of course only you can know how you are feeling, and only you can decide when things are too much for you—has been a traditional pastime in the UK for just over a century. In 1911 David Lloyd George, the Liberal chancellor of the exchequer at the time, was instrumental in the passage of the National Insurance Act 1911. This provided a system of national insurance for people in employment to cover the risks of illness and unemployment. It was funded by contributions from the employee, their employer and the state.[1]

In the case of sickness benefits workers paid 4d a week to the scheme, their employer 3d, and 2d was added from general taxation—what Lloyd George termed 'ninepence for fourpence'. In times of sickness individuals could claim 10 shillings per week for the first thirteen weeks of absence, and 5 shillings per week for the next thirteen weeks. Although it was a state scheme, it was administered by 'approved societies'—organisations registered under the Act and generally operated by 'Friendly Societies', trade unions and insurance companies—which had some latitude in its administration. The scheme also facilitated access to treatment from 'panel' doctors, who had a treatment role but also provided the initial sickness certification.

Early attempts at gatekeeping access to benefit were largely ineffective. The first benefits under the 1911 Act were paid in January 1913. Within eight months there was alarm that payments were considerably greater than those that had been predicted by the actuaries—the Friendlies were proving too friendly. As early as 1914, an inquiry was formed, chaired by Sir Claud Schuster,[i] to 'enquire into and report upon the alleged excessive claims' of the sickness benefits scheme.[2] As the inquiry heard evidence over the subsequent six months, various dilemmas became clear.

There was no universal understanding about what 'incapacity for work' actually meant, nor the extent to which it should relate to the member's actual job, versus a more notional concept of what 'work' might mean. This is another example of ambiguity as to exactly where the bar is set by ostensibly objective assessments about capacity for work. We have acknowledged the challenge of deciding, and defining, in any consistent way how much hardship we would expect claimants to endure in order to work—what we might call the Douglas Bader conundrum. Now it seems that establishing exactly what is taken to constitute work opens another can of worms.

---

[i] Schuster was not distinguished as a student nor subsequently as a barrister but was the consummate civil servant, acting as secretary to several committees and going on to be the longest-serving permanent secretary to the Lord Chancellor's Office, now the Ministry of Justice (a post he held for 29 years). It was his appointment as chief registrar of the friendly societies that placed him on the relevant committee and, soon after, as the chair of the inquiry into their effectiveness.

The inquiry report noted that doctors were inconsistent in their approach. Sometimes they might write misleading information on certificates in an effort to protect the patient's confidence; elsewhere they were pruriently obsessed with conditions that transgressed the social mores of the time, such as sexually transmitted disease or the health problems of unmarried pregnant women. The inquiry committee struggled with how to ensure the scheme be compliant with the legal requirement—created by the 1911 Act—that conditions arising from 'misconduct' should not be insured. At that time there would have been no aversion to writing the kind of report that Dame Carol Black would be asked to provide a century later.

The inquiry also noted that the scheme had created moral hazards for doctors. There was a suspicion that some panel doctors were quite happy to issue certificates readily, as that way they would attract more patients; they were paid on a capitation basis, in other words according to how many patients they had on their books. The conflict of interest arising from sickness schemes requiring certification by doctors was already becoming apparent. In a fairly weak attempt at resolving this conflict, the report attempted an appeal to the doctors' conscience to be mindful of the greater good. It urged that 'A regard for the interest of the patient, therefore, involves a duty to see that the undeserving do not receive benefit to the detriment of the deserving.'[3]

In subsequent years there was progressively more stringent government oversight over the societies administering sickness benefits. Guidance was issued about claims assessment, claimants accepted onto the scheme were visited at home by 'sick visitors' with a view to detecting malingerers, and questionable cases were increasingly referred to regional medical officers for adjudication.[4] The system became ever more bureaucratic and costly in its own right. The 'Friendly Societies' of the 1911 Act established an unhappy prototype for all sickness benefit schemes that would follow. Cost control was poor, so the amounts being paid out were well in excess of what had been forecast and budgeted for. As sickness levels continued to rise, seemingly unstoppably, there was a moral panic and increasingly desperate measures were used in an effort to keep a lid on things. The medical assessment process became more and more convoluted as local panel doctors referred ever growing numbers of contentious cases to the regional medical officers. Eventually, those administering the scheme resorted to a policing approach—sick visitors being the covert surveillance teams of their day—rather than relying solely on medical assessments. An instrument intended to improve the efficiency with which alms were delivered to the sick instead had the effect in practice of improving the flow of resources to a burgeoning administering bureaucracy.

Despite all the omens that using doctors as gatekeepers for sickness benefit schemes was a thoroughly bad idea, thirty-five years after the 1911 Act Beveridge unimaginatively used the same mechanism as a vital moving part in the machinery of the new welfare state. The practice of using doctors to certify claimants for sickness benefits was designed into the blueprints of the late 1940s. Within the newly created National Health Service, family doctors were required to issue sick certificates for the Ministry of National Insurance. The dream was that, by making treatments widely available and so making people healthier, in concert with a gatekeeping mechanism to prevent unnecessary sickness absence, the National Health Service might even pay its own way by improving the gross domestic product.[ii]

[ii] Beveridge believed that early treatment of diseases, once healthcare was widely and freely available, would improve productivity and be more cost-effective in the long run. His 1942 report (p. 105) estimated that Health Service expenditure would not rise over 20 years, 'it being assumed that there will actually be some development of the service, and as a conse-

The idea that a worker needed the writ of their doctor in order to legitimise their withdrawal from work had become an unquestioned meme during the decades that had elapsed since the first National Insurance Act. Those who colluded in the fantasy that this was something that doctors could do effectively, and who designed it into the infrastructure of the new welfare state, provided no evidence to support their belief. They could not, because what evidence had amassed since 1911 undermined their case.

It was an article of faith rather than of reason, and one that managed to endure because the policy-makers of the era continued to hold simplistic beliefs about the nature of illness and sickness. They believed that both were invariably and simply the consequence of disease. From this stemmed their confidence that, as the NHS got to grips with treating the backlog of disease they believed had accumulated in the era prior to socialised healthcare, so illness and sickness would begin to disappear. This way of thinking also cemented in their minds the idea that doctors were the ideal sickness assessors, being the experts in disease detection.

---

quence of this development a reduction in the number of cases requiring it.' One of his mistakes was to believe that the demand for healthcare was finite and that, once the 'backlog' of disease had been treated, demand would fall. Of course, in practice patients and their doctors will conspire to create new problems when old ones have been solved, and the demand for healthcare is infinite. In 1945 Minister of Health Nye Bevan estimated the cost of the new service at £145 million per year; he later had to tell his Cabinet colleagues that the cost forecast for 1949–50, the second year of operation, was £330 million. By 1951 it was necessary to introduce prescription charges for dental care and spectacles; Bevan resigned in protest. See HMG (December 1945), Cabinet briefing paper. 'Proposals for a National Health Service. A Memorandum by the Minister of Health'; and HMG (December 1948), Cabinet briefing paper. 'The National Health Service. A Memorandum by the Minister of Health'.

Whilst remarkable and foresighted in many ways, the father of the welfare state was by no means infallible. Beveridge's insinuation that the long-term unemployed should be castrated will have struck many as distasteful, even allowing for the attitudes of the era.[5] He was not a popular Cabinet member; the wartime minister of labour, Ernest Bevin, could not abide the prospect of working with him.[6] Although Beveridge wanted to be in the Labour Ministry, organising manpower on the Home Front, Bevin saw to it that he was sent to work on an inquiry into social insurance—a move that fortuitously culminated in the Beveridge Report.[7]

In his obituary, the journalist Kingsley Martin depicted Beveridge as lonely and despotic.[8] The accounts of his contemporaries depict him as more of a technocrat, with an excessively administrative perspective, than someone with a well-nuanced emotional intelligence or sense of the human condition. This seems to have given him a naively mechanical perspective on the doctor–patient relationship, in keeping with the times but also his personality. If he had had a greater sense of how complex and subtle this relationship can be, more understanding of how illness often has nothing to do with disease, and greater awareness of the problems that had bedevilled earlier attempts at certification, then he might have given more careful thought as to whether it was sensible to ask doctors to certify their patients' sickness. As it was, he unthinkingly repeated Lloyd George's mistake.

To make matters worse, not only were the policy-makers ignorant about the real nature of doctoring, but their relationships with the doctors were so poor that there was little opportunity for the politicians to be enlightened. Communications between the British Medical Association (the body representing the doctors) and the Ministry of Health were bitter; it was scarcely an environment of constructive collaboration.[9] Doctors intensely disliked the prospect of becoming employees of the state, and the proposals for a new national health service were likened to something that the Nazis might have approved of.[iii]

Hence, the creation of the new system was in the teeth of fierce opposition from doctors, not with their involvement and counsel. In a 1948 poll, just 4,735 out of 45,549 doctors supported the National Health Service.[10] Labour's minister for health, the Welshman Nye Bevan, famously admitted that he had 'stuffed their mouths with gold' in order to broker a deal between the BMA and the Health Ministry after eighteen months of wrangling.[iv]

Some sense of how things were likely to unfold was clear as early as 1946, just as it had been so soon after the 1911 National Insurance Act. History was rhyming as the mistakes were repeated. A BMA report titled 'The British Medical Association and the National Health Service Bill' contained the following passage:

> For the medical profession to be converted into a technical branch of central or local government would be disastrous both to medicine and to the public it serves. The doctor's primary loyalty and responsibility should be to his patient. The interest of the public demands that he should be free—as civil servants and local government officers cannot be—to act, to speak and to write on professional matters according to the dictates of his conscience, unhampered by interference from above. He should never be required, or be in a position to be required, to modify his standards of medical certification at the

---

[iii] Dr Alfred Cox described the proposed health service in 1946 as 'the first step, and a big one, towards National Socialism as practised in Germany'. *BMJ*, Vol. 1, Issue 4448, 541–543 (1946). 'Correspondence: The Health Service Bill'.

[iv] This was actually in relation to the contract with hospital consultants rather than general practitioners, but it is illustrative of the overall state of negotiations between government and doctors about the new service.

behest of the State, however concerned the State may be with the solvency of a Social Security Fund. This independence of professional judgment and responsibility of action, evolved over the centuries, is inconsistent with the conception of the doctor as a civil servant or local government officer, whose first loyalty would be to his employing body. Valuable though these forms of organization and control are in many fields of human activity, they would be fatal to the personal doctor-patient relationship which lies at the heart of good medicine. The doctor should be the patient's doctor and not the Government's doctor.[11]

It should have been fairly clear from the outset that the state's putative sickness police disliked their new masters, empathised with patients and were going to prove timorous officers. Embroiling them yet further in the politics of sickness, deaf to their protestations, was bound to end in tears. The error of the central planners was to continue to assume, in the face of all contradictory evidence to date, that the doctors' skills in diagnosing and treating disease were somehow transferable to the assessment and management of sickness.

7

PARADISE LOST

The postwar Attlee government was pledged to creating a 'New Jerusalem' at a time when the nation's finances had been exhausted by the exertions of war.[i] Industrial sickness absence was viewed as a threat to building this utopia. There was a desire to believe that the threat could be neutralised through a combination of healthcare provision and sickness certification.

Certainly the promise of improving availability of healthcare was fulfilled. The explosion in medical treatment since the creation of the National Health Service has been dramatic. Astounding technological advancements have been made and the NHS has facilitated their distribution, irrespective of the individual's ability to pay. This period has seen antibiotics, coronary artery stenting, treatment for high blood pressure and diabetes,

---

[i] The New Jerusalem epithet derives from a speech given in Scarborough in 1951 by Labour leader Clement Attlee, to launch the party's manifesto for that year's general election campaign. It ended with an extract from William Blake's *And did those feet in ancient time*. The video can be found online at https://www.youtube.com/watch?v=RNcX_t_AuVA [accessed

minimally invasive surgery and replacement of failing organs with artificial or donated ones. An orthopaedic surgeon named Austin T. Moore performed the first metallic hip replacement in 1940 (although there had been a heroic earlier attempt by Themistocles Gluck in 1891 using ivory, plaster of Paris and glue). Now 1.3 per cent of Britons possess a hip that is not their own.[1]

Knees, ankles, shoulders, elbows and wrists can all now be replaced, as can major blood vessels and organs for that matter. Developments in anaesthesia have made complex, lengthy surgical procedures viable when previously they would have been unbearable, fatal or both. In cancer medicine, surgical techniques have been refined and non-surgical treatments such as chemotherapy, radiotherapy and hormone therapy developed. We are entering the era of personalised cancer care, in which treatments are selected according to the genetic makeup of an individual patient and their tumour; monoclonal antibodies, which target specific proteins on cancer cells, are being used to delivery chemotherapy agents with astonishing selectivity. The human genome has been sequenced and gene therapy for some heritable diseases has become a reality.

The Attlee cabinet envisaged a fairer, more prosperous country with accessible healthcare and better teeth. By and large, that is what it got. Its aspirations to drive down sickness absence and improve the national wealth were not entirely fanciful, even if the omens of 1911 were not encouraging.[ii] Perhaps the new service's

---

13 November 2016]. Whilst the text is rousing the delivery is surprisingly underwhelming, even accounting for the tastes of 1951. Attlee is widely regarded as one of the most effective prime ministers Britain has had. Nevertheless this speech brings to mind Churchill's alleged witticism at Attlee's expense: 'A modest man with much to be modest about.'

[ii] Two assumptions underpinned the belief that the NHS could be a net contributor to GDP. First, it was assumed that the costs of the new service

sheer scale of ambition would mean it could succeed in eradicating sickness where earlier, small-scale attempts had failed?

The short answer is no. Attempts were made to measure trends in sickness absence during the post-war decades and the news was quickly disappointing. The NHS was just a teenager in 1962 when Health Minister Enoch Powell described as a fallacy the notion that improving the nation's health would necessarily and infinitely improve its wealth (in part through reducing industrial absenteeism).[iii/2] The statistics bore him out: despite enormous expenditure on the new health service, the number of people out of work—not paying taxes, and drawing from the benefits system—had been steadily going up, not down. In the fifteen years between 1949 and 1964, the Annual Reports of the Ministry of Pensions and National Insurance recorded a steady rise in sickness rates. On average there were 134,000 new claims for sickness benefit per week in 1949, and by 1964 this figure had risen by 29 per cent to 173,000 new claims per week. A 1965

---

could be constrained (see Chapter 6). The second assumption was that the service would generate a return on investment by reducing rates of industrial absenteeism. The hope that the NHS would represent a saving for the exchequer, through this combination of cost control and improved productivity, persisted for some years. In 1956 the Guillebaud Committee (an inquiry that had been formed to investigate the cost of the NHS) concluded that the health service would be 'a wealth-producing as well as a health producing service'.

[iii] In his lecture Powell refuted both of the assumptions underpinning the idea that the NHS could pay its own way. He described Beveridge's prediction that costs would not rise as a 'miscalculation of sublime dimensions', because in reality the demand for healthcare is infinite. Second, he observed that sickness rates had not fallen as predicted. Powell was not arguing against the Health Service per se, but that the justification for it should be acknowledged as moral and not financial. It remains true that,

academic paper by the renowned epidemiologist Professor Jerry Morris noted:

> During this period of advancing medical knowledge, improving standards of living and changing pattern of disease, there was a substantial fall in death rates at all ages under about 55, but no reduction in 'sickness absence' ... The situation is similar in organizations like the Metropolitan Police or the Post Office.[3]

A conundrum was presented. Those metrics which provided some insight into society's biology, such as the prevalence of particular diseases and premature death rates, were improving— yet worker presenteeism was not. By any objective measure people's physical health was improving, yet they were increasingly likely to take time off work. Why?

An occupational physician, Peter Taylor, found an intriguing clue. His research papers were periodically published by the *British Medical Journal* in the late 1960s. Taylor was the medical officer for the Shell refinery in Essex. Fortunately for us, if not for the employees, meticulous records of sickness absence and even lateness had been kept for 1,350 workers since the end of the war. Between 1949 and 1964 the percentage of working days lost to sickness absence increased fairly steadily from 2.97% to 3.89%, an increase of 31% and very similar to that described by Morris over the same time span.[4]

---

fundamentally, the electorate expects the NHS to provide care, not return-on-investment. Periodically during its history there have been proposals to prioritise the healthcare needs of working-age people, on the grounds that the sooner they have resumed work, the sooner they will begin paying tax again. However, these are quietly sidelined when the political ramifications of an economics-first approach to the NHS are considered: that the needs of certain demographics, such as the elderly, would need to be deprioritised.

What was particularly interesting about Taylor's research was that, because data was captured over such a long period, it was possible to reach conclusions about the way sickness behaviour was changing over time. It had long been known that younger men tended to have more frequent periods of sickness than older men. What had not yet been clear was whether they would grow out of it, or whether there were true generational differences. Taylor's work showed that this new generation of young men were recalcitrant: they continued their habit of poor attendance into their middle age. There was something significantly different from one generation to the next in terms of their propensity to take sick leave. Some fundamental social change was afoot. Despite all the improvements in healthcare, despite being richer, and despite having better working conditions, the postwar generation was taking much more time off work.

If the 1950s and 1960s were a disappointment for those who had hoped to see industrial absenteeism disappear as a problem, the 1970s and 1980s were a time when industrial relations were dysfunctional to a point that threatened systemic collapse of the economy. Measures such as the three-day week, a loan from the International Monetary Fund and radical reforms to trades union legislation were all introduced during this period. Sickness became an intensely political issue since government, desperate to persuade the electorate that matters were in hand and that the economy was not collapsing, felt that it was better to pretend that swathes of people had bizarrely become sick than to admit that the economy was collapsing. To achieve this they resorted to bribery.

Throughout these decades there were progressive increases in the monetary value of sickness benefits.[5] Prime Minister Margaret Thatcher made no fewer than seventeen changes to out-of-work benefits during her time in office. Her government urged doctors to deem workers who had been made unemployed eligible for sickness benefits, rather than leaving them to claim the dole.[iv] The number of sick workers rose by 40 per cent between 1985 and 1990, reducing the unemployment count by 400,000. In 1977 a survey found that 4 per cent of 59-year-old women had a chronic health problem impairing their ability to work; ten years later this figure had risen to 21 per cent.[6]

This widening of the gap between sickness benefits and other out-of-work benefits was a political tactic, designed to encourage the newly unemployed to apply for sickness benefit rather than unemployment benefit. The government's blushes were to be spared by artificially massaging down the unemployment statistics. Various high-profile politicians who inherited the legacy of this deplorably cynical policy—including former Labour Prime Minister Tony Blair, and former Tory Chancellor of the Exchequer George Osborne—have admitted as much, generally once out of office, as an aside in the memoirs.[7] Unsurprisingly, it is otherwise rarely discussed by them. Osborne has been one notable exception, remarking in 2013 while still serving as chancellor that the Thatcher government's actions had been 'quick-fix politics of the worst kind.'[v]

It was a sorry episode in our political and industrial history that has come to be seen as a public health disaster, still rippling

---

[iv] A former colleague who was practicing as a GP at the time in the north of England recalls his astonishment and anger on receiving such policy circulars.

[v] Speaking to a group of supermarket workers, whilst attempting to defend the coalition government's welfare reforms, Osborne said: 'Governments of all colours let too many unemployed people get parked on disability benefits, and told they'd never work again. Why? Because people on disability benefits don't get counted in unemployment figures that could embarrass politicians.' (*The Guardian*, 'Osborne distances himself from Thatcher's legacy'.)

across the generations, as much as an economic one. Research in
the twenty-first century, especially that commissioned as part of
the Blair government's 'Health, Work and Wellbeing' strategy,
has revealed quite how dangerous long-term economic inactivity
is to human health and longevity.[8] Social policy that acted to
incentivise long-term withdrawal from the labour market was as
bad for the national health as it was for the national wealth.
People who have been out of work for extended periods of time
are at risk of never returning, and the probability of this increases
the longer the period in which they are workless and becoming
deconditioned.[9] Absentees who have been away from work for
two years are more likely to die or retire than to return to
work.[10] That, in turn, poses a fiscal double whammy for the
exchequer—a lifetime of lost tax receipts, and of benefit payments in perpetuity.

The short-term benefit of such chicanery was political and
favourable to the schemers, who could simultaneously manipulate
the unemployment figures whilst portraying themselves as compassionate towards the sick. But the long-term effects were
human, economic and profoundly negative: this was treasonous
realpolitik. In some families it had the consequence of marginal-
ising two or even three generations, already desperate and vulnerable, from gainful employment, and from the opportunity for
social mobility that this would otherwise have brought. It also
had the particularly undesirable side-effect of hardening public
attitudes to sickness benefit claimants as a whole. Those who
truly were unemployable by virtue of their ill health came to be
stigmatised alongside those who had no place being on sickness
benefit and who had merely exercised a convenient choice presented to them by the politicians of the day.

Sickness levels steadily increased throughout the forty-five
years that followed the launch of the National Health Service,
reaching a zenith in the mid-90s.[11] But sickness had not been

properly acknowledged as a problem, because it did not fit conveniently with the political narrative of successive governments. For the social engineers of the immediate postwar years, highlighting the issue would have implied either that attempts at improving health were futile, or that the new generation was increasingly selfish in how much hardship it would endure before it was willing to be a burden to others. Either explanation subverted their ideal of a New Jerusalem. For their successors, sickness offered an opportunity for creative accounting—relabelling the unemployed as the sick was politically expedient. There was nothing to be gained by drawing attention to the growing problem of 'sickness', and so governments remained wilfully blind. Obstinacy and self-interest prevailed for decades.

By 1995 expenditure on state sickness benefits had ballooned to be approximately nine times greater in real terms than it had been in the mid-1950s.[12] The scale of the problem was such that it was now simply unavoidable. John Major, then prime minister, remarked in 1993, 'Frankly, it beggars belief that so many more people have suddenly become invalids, especially at a time when the health of the population has improved.'[13] The picture since that time has been one of progressive tightening of sickness benefits, in particular with the introduction of the Work Capability Assessment in 2008 as a means of governing access to Employment and Support Allowance.[14] Such attempts at reform became more urgent during the recessionary years after the 2008 financial crisis and the associated pressure to curb welfare spending. In 2010 the government published its white paper 'Universal Credit: welfare that works', proposing reforms to the existing labyrinthine benefits system and in particular a cap on the total amount payable to any given household.[15]

The percentage of the adult population in receipt of state sickness benefits decreased slightly from 6.5 per cent at the time of the Major government to 5 per cent in 2016. But this is anaemic progress for a first-world nation with a predominantly service-sector economy, world-leading health and safety statutes and a national health service. New Jerusalem we are not, even if we are no longer the sick man of Europe either. In its 2016 'Welfare Trends Report', the Office for Budget Responsibility forecast that the government's sickness reforms appeared to be running out of steam and that there was likely to be little change in the percentage of people receiving benefit within the next five years at least.[16]

Sickness levels also fell amongst the employed between 1993 and 2013 (claimant figures for state sickness benefits being a marker of sickness amongst the unemployed). The decline largely matches that seen in the sickness rate of the unemployed over the same period: of approximately a third to a quarter. This is apparent in statistics from the Labour Force Survey and from industry surveys such as those commissioned by the Confederation of British Industry and the Chartered Institute of Personnel and Development. The CBI's 'Absence and Workplace Health' 2013 employer survey found that absence had reduced by about a quarter since the 1980s to a 'record low' of 2.3 per cent.[17]

Whilst sickness absence amongst workers has been gradually reducing in the new millennium, there was a notable inflexion point—where rates fell noticeably—around the time of what is now being called the 'great recession' of 2008–9. Sickness rates fell successively for the subsequent four years, an unusually sustained period to see a consistent reduction in absenteeism. The Office for National Statistics' 2016 analysis of sickness absence in the labour market summarised the situation thus: 'Since 2003, there has been a general decline in the number of days lost to sickness absence, particularly during the economic downturn. Sickness absence fell to a low of 131.7 million days in 2013 but there were increases in 2014 and 2015.'[18] The drivers of sickness are complex and multi-factorial, but a heightened fear of job loss—or greater appreciation for the offer of work, depending on your perspective—in recessionary periods seems to play a significant role.

Whereas numbers of claimants for state sickness benefits are fairly definite, almost any measure of employee absence is likely to underestimate the scale of the problem. It is more likely that an absence will be forgotten by an employee subsequently asked to take part in a survey such as the ONS Labour Force Survey, or will not be recorded by their employer, than that someone would recall an absence in error, or be marked absent on a day they were actually at work. There are companies providing 'Day One' sickness absence services that take calls from employees reporting themselves sick, in order to record all sickness absences on behalf of client organisations. As this is their stock in trade, they record sickness absence data more consistently than the line managers of those companies are themselves able to. Anecdotally, the experience of such Day One companies, as reported to me, is that true sickness absence levels run approximately 20 per cent higher than is suggested by surveys such as those of the CBI—meaning that sickness absence is more likely to be in the region of 2.8 per cent than the 2.3 per cent suggested in 2013 by the CBI.

The record-keepers at Peter Taylor's Shell refinery were similarly fastidious. There the information was captured through employees having to manually punch their clock cards on arrival at and departure from work. His data is very likely to represent the true extent of sickness at that time. The remarkable thing is that the current level of sickness amongst the employed, probably around 2.8 per cent, is not so very different from that recorded amongst the workforce at the Shell refinery in 1949: 3 per cent.

At that stage the NHS was only just embarking on its mission to spend vast sums of money with the ambition of radically improving the nation's health and tackling the scourge of industrial absenteeism. We haven't come very far. Sickness rates remain stubbornly high compared with those of 1948, bearing in mind how much healthcare has improved and how much safer the workplace has become. It seems that social phenomena such as political gamesmanship, industrial unrest and economic crisis have much greater influence on the course of sickness within society than doctors wielding pens.

8

DISEASE INSPECTORS

The architects of the welfare state were concerned, amongst other things, with designing mechanisms to constrain the extent of industrial sickness in their New Jerusalem. 'Genuine' sickness was naively conceptualised as simply the result of human mechanical malfunction: disease. Naturally the assumption that flowed from this was that doctors, as the technicians trained in detecting disease—human biological faults—were therefore the people to validate claims to sickness. This would be in much the same way as vehicle engineers might assess the roadworthiness of a car on behalf of the Ministry of Transport, or a vet might insert their arm elbow-deep into a cow's rectum on behalf of a concerned farmer.

Neither the vehicle inspector nor the vet can question their patient about their symptoms. Sickness claimants can speak, but the people who advocate for sickness assessments are unlikely to see that as an advantage. They want people whom they fear are aspiring scroungers to be quite literally inspected and vetted, not doctored. For them, the individual is an Economic Man or Woman and therefore their account is not to be trusted. They would prefer their sickness police to be a little less Dr Finlay and more in the manner of the Stasi. In such people's eyes, an assessor who speaks to the claimant and accepts their story at face value is a fool not to have realised that they have broken the cardinal (but unspoken) rule of the game: they cannot believe a word they are told. One of the most common complaints from sickness assessments organised by employers is that the assessor is merely repeating what the individual has already said to them directly, as though it is a surprise that the employee has managed at least to be consistent with their story, whether it is real or fictitious.

Did the people who designed the welfare state have a similar expectation that doctors undertaking sickness assessments should fulfil an interrogatory, forensic function—quite at odds with the trusting and sympathetic role of the doctor in their ordinary therapeutic setting? Archibald Cronin's 1937 novel *The Citadel* would suggest so.[1] It tells the story of Dr Andrew Manson, who begins his working life as a novice doctor in the Welsh valleys. Whilst in Wales, Manson takes a job with the Miners' Medical Aid scheme in the fictional village of Aberalaw. Later he moves to London and establishes a practice in Harley Street, indulging hypochondriacs with expensive placebo remedies.

The novel was largely autobiographical, since Cronin himself had first practiced medicine in the valleys and subsequently in Harley Street. He had also worked with a Miners' Medical Aid scheme—the Tredegar Medical Aid Society—alongside a certain Nye Bevan, who was a trade union official in the area at the time. When Bevan later became health minister in Attlee's postwar government, it was the Tredegar Medical Aid Society that provided the small-scale model for his new National Health Service. The novel written by his erstwhile medical colleague was the literary expression of the same dream. *The Citadel* is a heavily laden morality tale, as propaganda is wont to be. It describes the wretched and perilous state of working people prior to socialised healthcare, and private practice is demonised as wicked and unethical. Manson is a moral hero, aghast at the poor quality of medical treatment available to the working people of the valleys and the lack of care on the part of those in positions of authority. He drifts from the path of righteousness during his time in London, but redeems himself by the conclusion of the novel.

The Citadel was hugely influential in the late 1930s. A 1938 Gallup poll found that the book 'impressed' more people than any other text save for the Bible, and it was reputed to have had a material effect on the result of the 1945 general election, which led to the founding of the NHS.[2] Given the extent to which Cronin and *The Citadel* are likely to have influenced Bevan's thinking about how the new health service should operate, what is interesting is the way in which Manson, a fictional model doctor, sets about the task of sickness certification. This is our strongest clue as to how Nye Bevan imagined that doctors should, in the real world, discharge their duty to certify.

Manson clearly sees certification as important and solely for a doctor to undertake. On his arrival in Wales he learns that the local doctor has been incapacitated by a severe stroke and that Dai Jenkins, a bumptious pharmacy dispenser, has become accustomed to working above his pay and grade. He has been holding surgeries over recent weeks, including the issuance of certificates using a doctor's stamp that the doctor's wife has made up for him. Manson makes it clear that from now on, only he— as the doctor—is to provide certificates for anyone.

He frets about the vast number of miners attending his clinic to demand a certificate, confiding in a colleague, 'I'm worried about the number of certificates I had to sign. Some of these chaps this morning looked to me quite capable of work'.[3] He frets, 'What can anyone think of a doctor who hands out certificates like cigarette coupons?'[4] The novel describes how 'Before afternoon his cogitation had forced him to an unpleasant decision. He could not, on any account, give a slack certificate. He went down to his evening surgery with an anxious yet determined line fixed between his brows.'[5] The following day's crowd of note-seekers are amazed at being examined by Dr Manson before he will provide a certificate, something that his careless predecessors never did. One man who is given a certificate is later enraged when he realises that it reads: '*This is to certify that Ben Chenkin is suffering from the effects of over indulgence in malt liquors but is perfectly fit to work.*'[6]

The Citadel is a fascinating glimpse into how those who designed the new health service thought about sickness certification. It was seen as a task that required much scientific knowledge, hence only something that was appropriate for doctors to do, and something that required them to adhere to high moral ideals. The model doctor was prepared to confront patients rather than to appease them, for the good of wider society. And the ills that patients brought to the surgery were the industrial diseases of the day—beat knee,[i] nystagmus,[ii] coal-miner's lung[iii]—conditions that Manson could confidently confirm or exclude with a suitably thorough approach to the examination of his patients.

Perhaps in the 1930s people were more prepared for their physicians to play roughly with them, and less inclined to com-

---

[i] Inflammation of a bursa (a fluid-filled pouch) at the front of the knee, normally caused by repeated kneeling. It is characterised by swelling, tenderness, redness and warmth.

[ii] A condition where there are involuntary, flitting movements of the eyes. Coal-miner's nystagmus was a compensable condition felt most likely to be due to a combination of work in poorly-lit conditions, adopting awkward head postures and the psychological distress of working in appalling conditions.

[iii] Scarring lung disease associated with prolonged inhalation of coal dust.

plain when they did so. But the attitudes and illnesses of twenty-first century Britons are light-years removed from those of the inhabitants of an interwar Welsh mining town. On internet forums, Manson's modern-day counterparts swap increasingly ridiculous examples of the demands asserted on primary care by some of today's patients: their aggressive sense of entitlement to particular tests, treatments, referrals and certificates, and their propensity to complain when these are met with any challenge.[iv] Interestingly, Cronin himself, sometimes portrayed as a champion of socialised medicine, envisaged the risks. He noted that a drawback of the Tredegar model was that 'with complete *carte blanche* in the way of medical attention the people were not sparing, by day or by night, in "fetching the doctor"'.[7] A malingerer's and hypochondriac's paradise.

Bevan hoped that Manson's bravery, forensic thoroughness and moral courage would be replicated in real life and on a wider scale by the doctors working within the new NHS. The idea that these attributes are prevalent amongst today's beleaguered general practitioners, or that they are able to refute claims to sickness merely through conducting a careful examination, is laughable.

Core to the doctrine of Bevan's socialised health service was the principle of free-at-the-point-of-access. After seventy years of persuasion that seeing a doctor is their entitlement rather than a privilege, the British populace has, unsurprisingly, come to see GPs as its state-sponsored servants (even if the contractual realities of the relationship between general practice and the NHS

[iv] One general practitioner recounted how a young female patient had expressed her worry that she was not able to drink more than 9 pints of lager, and therefore unable to keep up with her peers on a long night out. She was seeking advice about how her alcohol tolerance could be improved. The doctor's response, that if he were to drink 9 pints of lager there was a good chance it would kill him, was not received as helpful.

are a little more nuanced). In tandem with the loss of deference to experts and the professions in what has been termed the 'post-trust age', this means that the respect and power afforded to GPs in Cronin's day has now all but evaporated.[8/v] In today's mistrusting society, campaign groups for whatever malady is flavour of the day will regularly demean the general practitioner. Their marketing typically proclaims that doctors working in primary care don't understand the condition in question very well, with the patronising suggestion that they would benefit from being better educated about it (normally by the self-same campaigners). It is not something that many doctors are brave enough to publicly complain about. They fear being charged with that most wounding of accusations that can be levelled against them: having a God complex.

The subtleties and imperfections of actual medical practice—making finely balanced decisions quickly and on the basis of imperfect information, with increasingly limited referral options—do not intrude into the certain world of the armchair experts. Take, for example, the dilemma of GPs being urged to suspect and treat sepsis early and aggressively, in the face of the simultaneous campaign for them to exercise restraint over the prescription of antibiotics, to spare the world a plague of antibiotic-resistant microbes.[9]

In contrast, life is largely black and white for the non-medical campaigners promoting their particular fixation. They remain

---

[v] This sentiment was succinctly conveyed by Tory politician Michael Gove during the Brexit referendum campaign when he famously declared to Sky News, after it was put to him that many prominent economists disagreed with his assessment of the economic risks of Brexit, that 'people in this country have had enough of experts'. It has also been identified as an important theme by Baroness O'Neill of Bengarve, widely regarded as Britain's most eminent living philosopher.

unshakeable in their conviction that they are under a duty to educate the dullard family doctors. That their efforts to do so pass
generally without murmur is testament to how society at large now
regards GPs. There is a prevalent view that, as a non-specialist,[vi]
the general practitioner is likely to be intellectually challenged.
The 'education' they receive from campaigners normally includes
the exhortation to refer more quickly to hospital consultants. The
latter have managed to retain more of their kudos thanks to their
specialist credentials, the patient's lack of familiarity with them,
and their proximity to impressive-looking technology—a perception satirised by GPs as that of 'clever doctors in shiny hospitals'.

The power balance between today's family doctor and their
patient is very different to that of Dr Manson, dismissing his
'scrimshanker' with a flea in their ear. Despite that, the figure of
Manson lives on in the minds of many who mourn his passing.
Admirers of this robust approach to dealing with patients consider it appropriate—so long as doctors are interacting with other
people. When it is these 'hardliners' themselves who are rendered
vulnerable by illness and in need of a physician, they invariably
would prefer it to be Dr Finlay rather than the Stasi making an
appearance. If they attended the surgery for advice and certification about their headache, stomach upset or backache, and were
bellowed back out of it on the grounds that the doctor could find
nothing wrong with them, they would be the very first to complain, for they are honest and trustworthy patients. Double standards are at play.

This cognitive dissonance of the hard-pressed line manager—
that doctors are to treat them with kid gloves when they seek

---

[vi] Terminology which enrages some GPs, who argue that whilst their spe-
cialism is not defined according to the particular organ system that they
treat, they are self-evidently specialists in primary care.

healthcare, but are to interrogate their employees—would require doctors to swap hats depending on the occasion. The role of the doctor would transform depending on whether they are operating in a therapeutic setting or in a sickness assessment—from trusting confidant to ruthless investigator. But this was only ever true in the minds of Archibald Cronin and Nye Bevan. The presumption that doctors ever could or would shape-shift in this way was a mistaken and silly one, for it is to fundamentally misunderstand the nature of the social contract between doctors and the public.

Certainly the medical regulator is very clear that there is no duality of this kind. Good medical practice is defined independent of context—no distinction is drawn according to whether it is a therapeutic encounter or a sickness assessment. The first and overriding principle is that the care of the patient is the doctor's first concern; no caveats are applied. Admittedly the need for 'care' may be less obvious in a sickness assessment where there is no therapeutic relationship. But even if the setting is one in which there is no hands-on treatment, undoubtedly there is at least the expectation that the individual always be treated courteously and in good faith. In other words, that they be given the benefit of the doubt.

Society expects that at all times its nurses act as Florence Nightingale, and its doctors as Dr Finlay. The social contract with healthcare professionals is unspoken and implicit, but at its core is the expectation of servitude. They are not to be uppity with those in their charge, but should take at face value what they are told, except perhaps in circumstances where what is being reported is patently untrue. Given the nature of the things that patients report, which relate to sensations of body and mind that only they can feel, this is rare. In the absence of incontrovertible evidence to disprove them, patients are to be believed.

One doctor who had been engaged in sickness assessments reflected on these points whilst presenting at a conference. He had assessed a man who maintained that he had severely restricted movements of his shoulders. Having confirmed from the man that he could not reach behind his back with his left hand, he asked whether he could do so with his right. When the man answered that he could not reach behind with that hand either, the doctor triumphantly enquired, "But then how would you wipe your behind?!" At that moment, he was struck by the realisation that this, surely, could not be the kind of silly, distasteful exchange—demeaning to the doctor, humiliating for a patient who might well not be able to wipe his behind—in which society wishes its healers to engage.

Aside from the ethical objections to doctors mounting their own Spanish Inquisition of note-seekers, there are other constraints on them when it comes to assessing sickness that were also wholly unappreciated by the Attlee government. For instance, the way doctors interact with patients is not comparable with the way that an MoT mechanic sets about jabbing their screwdriver into a rusty chassis, nor with an episode of *All Creatures Great and Small*. What tools physicians do have in their kitbag are useful when applied in the therapeutic setting they were designed for: helping to identify and treat illness, and to alleviate distress. They are largely useless, and sometimes even unhelpful, when misapplied to a forensic setting.

Most importantly, the belief that 'true' sickness was invariably a consequence of disease, and that doctors—as disease inspectors—were therefore the best people to assess it, was incorrect even then. This is even more the case in an age where the major health issues afflicting Western society are illnesses, existing in the absence of any demonstrable disease process,[vii] and where the

---

[vii] As Dame Carol Black's 2008 'Working for a Healthier Tomorrow' report observes, the proportion of incapacity benefit claimants whose claim was

concept of mental illness especially is widely promoted.[viii] The Dr Mansons of today see very little beat knee or 'stagmus, but they do see a great many illness syndromes where they are wholly reliant on what the patient reports rather than what they can detect or test for directly. This includes phenomena such as stress, anxiety, depression, chronic fatigue syndrome, back pain, irritable bowel syndrome and fibromyalgia syndrome. In totality these represent the lion's share of the workload of the modern-day GP and occupational physician.

Although sickness rates crept inexorably upwards in the latter part of the twentieth century (post-1948), this was not as a result of people becoming steadily more diseased; we would have to ask some searching questions of the National Health Service if they had. Fluctuations in sickness do not correlate with changes in disease patterns and cannot be explained by them. The belief that disease and sickness are siblings could not be further from the truth. There is some level of relationship—at least some sickness is biologically determined—but the evidence currently available is that they are fairly distant cousins.

A dispassionate look at the evidence leads to an inevitable conclusion. Whatever the factors that cause sickness may be, they

---

as a result of a mental health problem rose from 26% to 41% within just 10 years (1996–2006). The World Health Organization has described depression as the leading global cause of disability.

[viii] Since the brain exists in a physical sense, its normal structure and function can be demonstrably disrupted; in other words it can become diseased. When it does we categorise the condition as a neurological disorder rather than a psychiatric one: for example, Alzheimer's disease or Parkinson's disease. Since the mind is not an organ that exists in a physical sense, nor can its malfunction: the mind cannot be diseased. Thus we always speak in terms of mental illness, and never mental disease.

are predominantly non-biological and are not effectively kept in check by doctors. Professor Jerry Morris began to speculate as much back in 1965, when he identified the paradox of rising sickness levels amongst a workforce whose health, where it could be measured objectively, was improving. He observed how closely the steady rise in sickness since 1950 had mirrored other social trends such as increases in consumer spending, crime, the birth rate and the number of people entering higher education.[10] Taken together, all these pieces of information showed that society was undergoing a fundamental change. Rising levels of sickness were part of a social revolution, not a medical phenomenon. The beguilingly simple belief that ill-health was the cause of sickness was simply not credible. Instead it has become irrefutable that cultural, social, financial, economic and political factors are overwhelmingly the main drivers of sickness. But what are these factors?

War in particular has strange effects on the national psyche and how individuals behave. Implacable political opponents begin to cooperate. At the outbreak of the First World War the major trade unions agreed with a government request to suspend the strike action that had been afflicting the country since 1910, known as 'The Great Unrest', so as to support the war effort.[11] People seemed to forget, or put aside, troubles that suddenly felt less vital. The Second World War was another period of collective hardship and individual peril. At certain points, such as the period when Hitler's plan for a seaborne invasion of England was imminent, there were real threats to the country's very survival as a sovereign state. The country endured but, by the end of the war, was grieving and destitute. The coffers had been exhausted and in 1946 Britain entered the Anglo-American Loan Agreement, which it would spend the next sixty years repaying to its ally. Rationing remained in force for a further eight years beyond Germany's surrender. Any sense of individual entitlement, such as it ever existed before the war, had been practically expunged from the national character by the end of it.

Few things influence suicide rates in a positive way, but the psychiatrist Andrew Malleson describes in *The Medical Run-Around* how suicide rates fell by 20–50 per cent in the combatant countries of the Second World War. There was a similarly significant fall in suicide rates—and indeed depressive illness—in Northern Ireland during the summer of 1969, following the outbreak of the Troubles; rates had been climbing for the preceding twenty-five-year period. Malleson contends that nothing seems to cheer people more than a good fight, which certainly seems more effective than psychiatric care in reducing the suicide rate.[12]

In times of conflict people are distracted from their personal battles—whether with their employer or their own psyche—by a new and more immediately threatening foe, in the shape of the Hun or a rival community. It is not difficult to see how an individual's sense of their own importance can be diminished when their nation-state is threatened with extinction, and in turn how their sense of obligation to endure hardship in the interests of the greater good would shift. It is difficult to be a prima donna in the midst of a blitz. Since sickness is heavily influenced by prevailing attitudes about how much hardship workers should have to bear in order to continue working, we might anticipate that war years would be periods of relatively low absenteeism.

Data about sickness absence during periods of major conflict is inevitably scant. Mass mobilisation of workers, widescale introduction of women into roles previously occupied by men, and civil disruption associated with the bombing of urban areas all made the collection and analysis of data during or from the Second World War very difficult. Similarly, comparison of pre- and post-war sickness rates is complicated by the radical transformation of social security in 1948.[13] However, we have one contemporaneous commentary, from Sir Henry Bashford, who was chief medical officer to the Post Office, and medical advisor to the Treasury in the later years of the war. In 1944 he observed that

> there is rather a paucity of available figures [about wartime sickness absence rates]. But if the 260,000 odd Post Office population is any sort of a barometer, there has not so far been evidence of any serious deterioration in health. In certain large cities, indeed, sick rates have been actually lower than in the three years immediately preceding the war. Amongst workers in other places, and particularly women workers[ix]—and particularly again in the more heavily bombed areas—there has been an increase.[14]

By the mid-1950s things were beginning to look very different. Rationing was lifted, the threat of extinction posed by hot war was receding into the national memory, the Cold War had yet to begin in earnest, and there was a newfound optimism in a scientific, better, safer and more comfortable future. Morris found it noteworthy that these social changes really took off around 1953. This year marked an inflexion point in each of the graphs plotting consumer spending, crime, birth rates and entry into higher education. He also remarked that, of these four graphs, it was consumer spending that most closely matched the graph of rising sickness levels.

[ix] This disparity had been noted by academics—and politicians—in the First War, and again was a source of concern in the Second. As commentators like Karlsson have critiqued, the explanation is likely to involve the fact that, despite women being expected to take on monotonous, exhausting work in munitions factories and the like, the social mores of the time—and the practical realities—meant that they were still not excused the lion's share of domestic and caring responsibilities. T. Karlsson, 'Gender differences in absence from work: Lessons from the two world wars', Institute for Evaluation of Labour Market and Education Policy, 2016, https://www.ifau.se/globalassets/pdf/se/2016/wp2016-26-gender-differences-in-absence-from-work.pdf [accessed 7 October 2018].

The connection is inescapable: as people became accustomed to a rising standard of living, their sense of entitlement began to grow, diminishing their sense of duty to work when feeling less able to do so. Whereas once someone might have tolerated 7.8 Jobs on our fantasy hardship scale, they might now only tolerate 6.2. This is a much more satisfactory explanation than the idea that people were inexplicably becoming more ill. Likewise, the social, political and economic circumstances of the last forty years also contextualise sickness trends better than any medical explanation. The steady creep in sickness levels amongst both the employed and the unemployed was becoming a substantial economic threat by the 1970s—but, for the reasons given in Chapter 7, political discourse was slow to admit this, and necessary reforms were delayed. From then onwards the country experienced a sequence of recessions—in the early 1980s, the early '90s and after the financial crisis of 2008—and irresistible economic forces began to assert themselves. In tandem with this, sickness levels have receded somewhat in the twenty-first century. Again, people's attitudes about how much hardship they may need to endure in order to remain in work began to harden; this time in the face of economic threats rather than military ones.

What is fascinating about these societal changes is that attitudes to illness itself were evolving. Views of what is and what is not a legitimate 'medical problem' change over time. Periodically all human lives inevitably entail disappointment, loss, physical hardship and mental suffering. When experiences accepted unthinkingly by one generation as an unchangeable and unavoidable part of life's rich tapestry are reformulated by the next as medical problems that might be solved, we can say that medicalisation has occurred. As societies become richer, and technology advances accordingly, the urge to medicalise becomes stronger. Rising levels of disposable income and industrialisation mean that better things can be bought, more easily, by ordinary people—cars, dishwashers, foreign holidays—so why not better health and 'wellbeing' too? Discomforts that were tolerated by preceding generations of workers come to be seen as intolerable because of the belief that medicine may be able to alleviate them.

This engenders an unfortunate combination of entitlement and diminished resilience. Whilst these are sometimes proposed as being defining traits of millennials, the society predominant as this generation has come of age is merely the culmination of an ongoing trend throughout the postwar years. In industrialised societies where healthcare becomes progressively more commoditised, while traditional cultural and religious beliefs that once fostered stoicism wane, people gradually lose their sense of self-reliance and their ability to cope with adversity. One of the expressions for this is a rising sickness rate—despite improvements in health as far as this can be objectively measured, for instance by rising life expectancy. This growing sickness is largely attributable to the 'new' illnesses that have been conceived, and stress-related absence from work is the apogee of this effect.

Those who believe that doctors should perform sickness certification on behalf of society tend to do so on the simplistic assumption that sickness is related to disease, and that it is culturally permissible for doctors to act as dispassionate disease inspectors when they interact with patients. They are woefully wrong on both counts. Most sickness has little if anything to do with disease, since modern society is quite prepared to accept that human suffering can exist in the absence of disease. The doctor who dismisses a claim to sickness on the grounds that they can find nothing 'objectively' wrong with the individual— i.e. they can find no disease—will find themselves in hot water, and learn not to do so again.

9

RELUCTANT GAMEKEEPERS

'Nie mój cyrk, nie moje małpy.'
Polish proverb ('Not my circus, not my monkeys.')

The power of the doctor's writ means they can be drawn into all kinds of squabbles, and their utterances then deployed for political gain. In 2015 there were concerns about the fitness of presidential candidate Donald J. Trump to assume the mantle of leader of the free world. His personal physician, Dr Harold Bornstein, provided a report intended to reassure the American electorate about Trump's vigour and rude health. It contained some suspiciously non-medical sounding hyperbole, describing his physical strength and stamina as 'extraordinary', his blood pressure as 'astonishingly excellent', and concluded that he would be the 'healthiest individual ever elected to the presidency'.[1]

Subsequently the two fell out over a breach of confidence committed by Dr Bornstein. He revealed to *The New York Times* that he had prescribed a hair growth promoter called Propecia® to his distinctively coiffured patient.[2] A couple of days later, one of Trump's former bodyguards made an unannounced visit to Dr

Bornstein's surgery to seize the president's medical records, and Trump reportedly severed contact with his doctor of thirty years. In retribution, Bornstein declared to the media that 'He dictated that whole letter. I didn't write that letter,' making some retrospective sense of grammar that had sounded more like the dialogue from *Bill and Ted's Excellent Adventure* than a medical report. Bornstein added, perhaps naively, 'I couldn't believe anybody was making a big deal out of a drug to grow his hair.'[3]

Normally, though, when doctors are being leant on it is to certify the presence rather than the absence of illness. In many jurisdictions around the world, police officers are prevented by law from going on strike. When labour relations are heated, one of the pressure valves available in other workforces—the option of withdrawing labour—is not available to the police. Predictably, the pressure finds its way out under other guises, co-ordinated days of mass sickness absence being one of these (so-called 'blue flu'). Further controls must therefore be applied by senior managers, such as the requirement to obtain a doctor's note for even a single day of absence—in other words, the removal of the right to self-certification. In Manitoba, in 1998, more than 100 officers truanted in protest at the suspension of a colleague. The requirement to obtain a certificate did not prove insurmountable for them. Fifty doctors who had issued notes were summoned before the Canadian province's College of Physicians and Surgeons to explain themselves.[4]

What do doctors think about finding themselves positioned between warring factions and used as pawns in this way? Blue flu is an extreme manifestation, but amongst note-seekers low-level disaffection and dissatisfaction with their employment is a frequent theme. In my experience, people who are enamoured with their job are less inclined to seek an exemption from it just because they are feeling less well than normal (experiencing, say, 1.2 Jobs of adversity). Researchers have canvassed the views of general practitioners and they are under few illusions as to their unsuitability for this particular aspect of their role. When teenagers predicted to achieve high A-Level grades are preparing their application to medical schools, they will have carefully prepared their stock answers as to why they wish to become doctors. An altruistic desire to help people, a strong sense of vocation and an opportunity to apply technology and the scientific method for the common good are all probable on the shortlist. A burning desire to be a judge for the Department of Work and Pensions or to arbitrate poisonous employment disputes is less likely to be cited. No doubt mentioning such aspirations would put an end to whatever chance the applicant might have had.

Unsurprisingly, it also does not emerge as an ambition during or after five or six years of medical training. One of the traits of people attracted to the caring professions is that they themselves may have some need to be needed. Whilst few people genuinely don't care whether they are liked, the theory that many doctors find it particularly hard not to be liked appears eminently plausible. They are probably different in this regard from police officers or fraud investigators, for example. This is not a personality type especially well-suited to confronting patients on behalf of the faceless spectre of the DWP.

When doctors are asked for their perspective, they report feeling coerced into an unsatisfactory process that is riven with inconsistencies, in exactly the way that the BMA argued they would be in 1911 and in 1948.[5] On the one hand, their professional bodies and the medical regulator emphasise how important it is for doctors working in primary care to make positive, enduring relationships with their patients—relationships which may need to be sustained for decades. The General Medical Council goes so far as to advise them, 'You must work in partnership with patients'.[6] On the other, they are also asked periodically to sit in judgment on these same patients, over their claims that they do not feel well enough to work. This bizarre curate's egg of a job has been described in oxymoronic terms as being a 'judgmental advocate'. Clearly, between these competing tensions, something has to give. Unsurprisingly, doctors are clear that they don't prioritise acting as a judge for the DWP, or for employers, over their concern to maintain a relationship with their patient.[7]

Many doctors are of the view—fairly, in my experience—that a great number of employers are neglectful of their employees. Or perhaps, more generously, at least neglectful of dealing with difficult employees. They view the sickness certification process as a means of inappropriately transferring responsibility for trying to keep people in work 'onto an [already] overstretched primary care service', a kind of medically mandated approach to work attendance.[8]

This may help to account for the finding of another study that some doctors even attempt deliberately to misuse or subvert the system. They do this by providing certificates as and when demanded by patients, and then writing vague or meaningless diagnoses on them, such as 'debility' or 'TALOIA'.[i] This same study contains the gems that 'acquiescence to every patient can ... be seen as a form of sabotage, rendering the gatekeeping role useless', and that some participants 'commented with satisfaction that the resulting statistics from certificates must be meaningless'. Whilst the po-faced may treat certification statistics with academic seriousness, evidently many of the doctors who provide them are ROFL.[ii]

It surely can't be surprising that there are doctors intent on sabotage. Doctors are unusual amongst the professions in that

---

[i] 'There's A Lot Of It About.' Examples from yesteryear include '*plumbum pendulum*' (swinging the lead) and 'GOK' (God Only Knows).
[ii] Rolling On Floor Laughing.

their working life is often conducted exclusively within, or at least contracting to, the National Health Service—a behemoth of 1.7 million people. According to data from the World Economic Forum, published by *Forbes*, the NHS was Europe's largest employer in 2015, and ranked number five in a list of the world's ten largest employers. Only the US Department of Defense, the People's Liberation Army of China, Walmart and McDonald's were larger. It certainly exceeded the Indian Railways and Indian Army, ranked at numbers eight and nine with their measly respective headcounts of 1.4 and 1.3 million employees.[9]

Working in one of the most sophisticated and emotionally demanding supply chains imaginable, in an organisation run by central planners in a manner not dissimilar to an East German supermarket, is demoralising for medical graduates in much the way that their predecessors predicted it would be in 1948.[iii] When its staff are asked about their experiences of working for the NHS, common themes of powerlessness, hopelessness and inertia emerge, as might be expected for a largely monopolistic employer of this size.[10] It is interesting to speculate on the morale of today's legal profession—perhaps the most obvious comparison in terms of academic entry requirements and remuneration—had its members been engulfed in a National Legal Service in the brave new world of 1948.

Doctors exasperated by working within such a monolithic and seemingly unaccountable institution might well have a distorted perspective about employers more generally.[iv] This bias is com-

---

iii The Department of Health's 2009 review of staff health describes bullying and harassment as 'deep-rooted cultural issues that are endemic in the NHS' (Boorman, 'NHS health and wellbeing review: interim report', p. 22).

iv Articles alleging that failed senior NHS managers have been re-employed elsewhere in the system after an unseemly brief purgatory abound in

pounded by the fact that patients are only liable to discuss their employment situation with their doctor when it is going particularly badly, and then in impassioned terms. Patients tend not to drop in to see their doctor to report how much they are enjoying their job and getting on with their manager. It is not fanciful, then, to suspect that certificating doctors may sometimes project their own dissatisfaction about their employment circumstances onto those of their patient. In this dynamic, issuing a certificate would represent a form of release, providing a small but real sense of having stuck it to the man. At least, it is difficult to attribute any other explanation to the actions of a French physician in Dunkirk, chastised by the local health authority for his generosity in providing 4,200 sick-notes over a four-month period, approximately fifty per day.[11]

The woeful lack of relevant training for doctors about the complex interactions between work and health—occupational health—has long been bemoaned. In one study, 63 per cent of general practitioners stated they had had no training whatsoever in sickness certification. For those who had, the average length of training throughout their entire career, as far as they could recall, had been 4.1 hours.[12] A different survey found that 70 per cent of GPs felt that the patient's judgement had to be relied upon: effectively a system of 'certification-on-demand'.[13] Interestingly the majority of doctors did not believe that further training was the answer, however. They felt that this would not resolve their con-

---

the press. One of the most high-profile NHS scandals, that of the Mid Staffordshire NHS Trust, resulted in a public inquiry (the Francis Report) in which a series of management failures were deemed to have contributed to 'appalling' standards of care and potentially hundreds of deaths. The chief executive of the Trust declined to give evidence to the inquiry on grounds of stress-related illness and was subsequently appointed as chief executive of an alcohol and addiction service. Cynthia Bower, who

cern that what they were being asked to do was a fundamentally inappropriate conflict of interest within their role.

Then there are the acute time pressures on the primary care consultation. The average length of a GP consultation is somewhere around 600 seconds.[14] Encouragingly, one study found that the duration of consultations is increasing by an average of 4.2 seconds per year, meaning that the fifteen-minute appointment might become a reality as soon as 2086. The study assessed the average consultation time in sixty-seven countries and found that the UK ranked twenty-ninth, behind countries including Peru, Bulgaria, Latvia, Poland and Croatia.[15] GPs can be forgiven for thinking that the odds are stacked against them, even if they are inclined to explore the complex factors that might underlie a patient's request for a sick-note. Not all these appointments will be purely for certification purposes, but a substantial amount of time is unarguably spent dealing with the administration of certification requests rather than on therapeutic work. Professor Max Kamien, an Australian doctor who estimates that he has issued 20,000 sick-notes during his career—and who has called for the abandonment of sickness certification as a costly waste of time—judges that '80 per cent of these so-called consultations are solely for the purpose of getting the sickness certificate.'[16]

---

had been chief executive of NHS West Midlands for 2 years before the scandal erupted, went on to become the first chief executive of the Care Quality Commission before having to resign that post after a Department of Health inquiry identified management failings in her new organisation. Sir David Nicholson, who had been chief executive of the Shropshire and Staffordshire Strategic Health Authority—responsible for the hospital—went on to become chief executive of NHS England. All this in the context of a scandal so great that Prime Minister Gordon Brown and Health Secretary Alan Johnson offered their personal apologies to those affected.

Statistics about the proportion of GP appointments where a sick-note is issued vary, and geography and demographics will play a part, but it is likely to be in the region of 10–35 per cent of cases.[17] On average, in England each month one certificate is issued for every forty-nine people aged between eighteen and sixty-five.[18] ONS data indicates that in 2016 the UK as a whole had 41.4 million people of 'traditional working age' (the very similar age band of sixteen to sixty-four).[19] If the NHS data for England is extrapolated—assuming similar rates of certification in the other home nations—this would equate to 845,386 certificates each month across the UK, or an astonishing 10.1 million certificates each year.[v] And this estimate excludes those issued to people who are under eighteen or over sixty-five. Enormous amounts of clinical time are spent—or, I would say, wasted—issuing these chits. This is a diversion that we can ill afford given that patients now have to wait an average of almost thirteen days for an appointment with a GP.[20] Some of them will have clinical needs much more pressing than those of the patients merely requiring the doctor's secretarial services in order to satisfy the DWP.

As if it were not bad enough to be asked to do something you don't feel it is appropriate or possible to do, to the detriment of the things you should be doing and already don't have time for, there is the threat of being reported to your professional regulator for doing so. Britons report doctors who have displeased them to the General Medical Council (GMC) in ever increasing numbers, particularly since the Shipman affair, after which it became the received wisdom that all doctors must be treated as

[v] This estimate excludes those over 65 who are still in work. ONS data for 2016 ('Five facts about … older people at work') was that 10.4% of over-65s remained in employment (1.19m people). If we assume similar rates of certification for these people as for the 18–65s, this is a further 24,286 sick-notes per month, or another 291,432 per year.

sociopaths in waiting.[vi] In the eight-year period between 2007 and 2015, there was an 81 per cent rise in the number of complaints made to the regulator by patients, from 3,615 to 6,547.[21] This is implausibly steep; it defies credibility that doctors had become almost twice as useless during such a short period of time. Instead, as with sickness rates, the explanation as to why complaints increased so sharply is more likely to entail sociocultural factors, and particularly patients' changing expectations of what their doctors are supposed to be doing for them.

As a regulator, the GMC has teeth, as well patients might expect. It has been delegated the statutory powers needed to censure doctors, to attach conditions to their practice, and to suspend or even erase them from the medical register. As such, it has the power to prevent doctors from earning a living in their chosen profession, in which—in order to qualify—they have invested at least five years of undergraduate training and, typically, a further

---

[vi] Dr Harold Shipman rose to notoriety as a mass murderer following his conviction at the outset of the new millennium, in January 2000, of having murdered 15 patients. Subsequent investigations suggested the true scale of his crimes could be in the region of 250 victims. Shipman was a murderer who happened to be a doctor, and who therefore had ease of access to means of killing people not available to most serial killers. Astonishingly, to this day he is the only British doctor ever to be convicted of murdering his patients. The day after Shipman's conviction the Secretary of State for Health, Alan Milburn, announced that there would be an independent inquiry. The resultant Shipman Inquiry—which ran until 2005, at a cost of £21 million—resulted in wide-ranging legal reforms to healthcare, especially the degree of oversight of doctors. It was as a result of the Shipman Inquiry that the current system of medical appraisal and re-licensing came into being. The Shipman scandal therefore represented a societal loss of innocence, a watershed moment that irrevocably changed the nature of the doctor-patient relationship in the UK.

five years of postgraduate study to become a general practitioner, or seven to nine years to become a hospital consultant. In 2015, seventy-two doctors were removed from the register, ninety-five were suspended from it, twenty-four had conditions attached to their practice, and 141 were issued warnings.[22]

Evidently, only a small proportion of patient complaints are both upheld and considered sufficiently serious to result in some significant impact on the concerned doctors' ability to ply their craft. But this is little consolation to those experiencing the misery of being subject to GMC processes, for whom the sword of Damocles can sometimes be suspended for a protracted period of months or even years. This has a stultifying effect on the physician's tendency to voice their honest opinion, as distinct from the one that is favourable to the patient. Doctors have a sense of self-preservation like anybody else and, unsurprisingly, being the subject of a complaint makes it much more likely that they will acquiesce to patient demands in the future. A survey of 7,926 doctors published in the *British Medical Journal* in 2015 found that 84.7 per cent of doctors who had had a recent complaint felt that they were now practicing more defensively. Fear of complaint can also encourage defensive practice even in the absence of actually receiving one. Almost 73 per cent of doctors with no previous complaint reported changing their practice simply after observing a colleague's experience of a complaint being made against them.[23]

In effect, the system—which purportedly restricts inappropriate access to sickness benefits—operates as follows. Graduates who have self-selected into a medical degree on the basis of altruism, and sometimes a need to be needed, are expected to confront inappropriate requests for certification from patients whom they will encounter repeatedly over many years, on behalf of a faceless bureaucracy, without thanks, and with approximately

600 seconds to do so on each occasion. At the same time, they are regularly reminded that they have a professional responsibility to maintain relationships with these same patients, potentially for decades. Their ability to earn a living depends on being licensed by the medical regulator, of whom they are fearful with some justification, yet they are expected to deny patients—who are reporting doctors to the regulator with unprecedented frequency—access to money and the preferential treatment that they may have been scheming to obtain. These doctors aren't trained in the task, to which their actual specialist area of competence—the detection and treatment of disease—is largely irrelevant. Predictably, they don't feel that it is an appropriate activity for them to undertake, and their response is typically to give the patient what they want or, for the more militant, to actively undermine the system itself.

The situation has been aptly summarised as one in which GPs perceive themselves as 'reluctant gatekeepers who know they can easily be circumvented by patients'. When I first encountered this quote, I misread the reference to gatekeepers as being to gamekeepers. It is an accidental but satisfying metaphor that I have appropriated for a chapter title. The browbeaten keeper seeks to protect the assets of an absent and unappreciative landlord from the plunder of people with whose predicament he can empathise—all the time fearing that some may be ready to cause him harm should he obstruct their pursuit of their quarry. Retreat to his lodge, venturing out occasionally to make a show of remonstrating a little with some of the less aggressive-looking poachers, seems like rational self-interest given the circumstances.

In private, at least, doctors have long conceded that they are largely passive observers when it comes to the charade that is sickness certification. In 1964 Dr Ranald Philip Handfield-Jones, one of the founding members of the Royal College of General

Practitioners,[vii] wrote in *The Lancet* that 'Examination by the doctor is usually a meaningless formality, since it is the patient who decides when he is fit for work.'[24] Much to the annoyance of many managers over many years, nothing has changed since.

[vii] Handfield-Jones practised in Haddenham, Buckinghamshire between 1954 and 1983. His *BMJ* obituary explains how times changed in that period: 'His first surgeries were held in the pub. They then moved to the back of the family house, where two rooms sufficed to provide waiting room, surgery, examination room, minor ops area, mini laboratory, and a dispensary ... After more than 20 years of twice daily surgeries, many house calls, and domiciliary obstetrics, he took on a partner and moved to the health centre that he had helped design and plan.' This is an example of the practical wisdom that the doctors of the period must have cultivated.

MEDICALISATION

10

THE LAND OF THE BLIND

Until as recently as the seventeenth century, there was little or no conception that symptoms might be symptomatic of anything. The patient's symptoms were themselves the condition. Not surprisingly, the treatments of the time were largely useless, because they were not informed by any scientific understanding of how the symptoms were caused. Perhaps occasionally, and by good fortune, the quacks[i] would chance upon a treatment that happened to ameliorate a symptom; but these were shots in the dark. By and large they tutted and blew their cheeks whilst nature took its course, perhaps applying cautery, poultices, leeches, cups and setons along the way. All of which generally hastened rather than delayed the demise of their patient.

Then, in 1676, the English physician Thomas Sydenham authored *Observationes mediciae* (Observations of Medicine).[1] Meticulous and recorded study of diseases meant that the mecha-

---

[i] From the Dutch word *quacksalver*, which once meant an amateur who healed with home remedies and in time came to be synonymous with 'charlatan'.

nisms by which they generated symptoms came to be better understood, and more effective treatments could be designed from first principles. Sydenham's revelation was that symptoms could signify an underlying disease process. As a result, physicians gradually learnt to treat pneumonia rather than catarrh, tuberculosis rather than consumption, coronary artery disease rather than angina, or auto-immune disease rather than rheumatism.

This was a quantum leap from interpreting illness as the punishment of vengeful deities, or as an imbalance between the four humours (blood, yellow bile, black bile and phlegm). It ushered in the golden age of medicine where, especially since the early twentieth century, astounding treatments for a range of diseases that would previously have been fatal—infections, cancers, vascular diseases—have become commonplace. It is not surprising that society came to have such extraordinary faith in the practitioners of these modern miracles. But this confidence in doctors is misplaced when they apply themselves to problems that exist in the absence of disease: when they attempt to treat illnesses for which there is no identifiable biological cause.

Many people believe that such situations are rare; that the patient whose symptoms remain unexplained despite all attempts at diagnosis is an unfortunate curiosity. In fact, the opposite is true. Only in a minority of patients is a causative disease process identified. The great majority of people who develop a symptom of whatever kind—headache, backache, bellyache, whatever—even those who consider their symptoms sufficiently serious for them to consult a doctor, will turn out not to have any identifiable disease to account for their symptoms. In one landmark study, researchers reviewed the records of 1,000 patients in a medical outpatient clinic, over a three-year period. They found that, of all the symptoms patients reported to their doctors, an underlying cause was never found in 84 per cent of cases.[2]

When doctors cannot identify a cause for a particular set of symptoms—which is most of the time—they are prone to cheat, by applying a label to them anyway. Patients like to think that their doctors know what is going on, so impressive-sounding syndromes (with names that in truth are purely descriptive) are correspondingly common. This is widely misinterpreted as implying that the cause of the condition is understood, or that it necessarily 'exists' in the tangible sense of a disease (like the fatty plaque of coronary artery disease or the scarred nervous tissue of multiple sclerosis), rather than solely as an experience that patients report (an illness). This is true for many of the afflictions of modern life, such as anxiety, depression, stress, chronic fatigue syndrome, fibromyalgia syndrome and irritable bowel syndrome.

To describe this process as diagnosis is to flatter. It is an exercise in pattern recognition and nomenclature rather than one of scientific insight into the causation. Paradoxically, the 'diagnosis' of these conditions requires first the confident exclusion of the presence of any disease that could cause similar symptoms. If such a disease had been detected, then that would be the diagnosis. Take a patient who is chronically tired—if it is established that the cause is an underactive thyroid gland, then hypothyroidism is their diagnosis, rather than chronic fatigue syndrome. Hence illnesses whose defining characteristic is that they exist in the absence of disease are referred to as diagnoses of exclusion.

The medical pioneers of yesteryear spent their lives searching for disease in order to make their diagnoses, because they were learning that these were the disorders they were most likely to be able to treat. Bizarrely, today's physicians spend most of their time seeking to confirm its absence in order to make theirs. But illnesses with little or no biological basis—at least, none that the best thinking and technology of the day can identify—prove a predictably hard nut for science to crack. Necessarily, the medics are then back to the tutting and educated guesswork of the pre-Sydenham days, rather than devising definitive cures in the way that is possible when a cause-and-effect relationship has been established. The various schools of thought about the causes of the condition are then free to bicker endlessly about the most appropriate treatment, with about as much acumen as royal physicians would once have employed arguing over the medical significance of the contents of the king's chamber pot.

Modern medicine and its practitioners earned their stripes in the pioneering days of the twentieth century, as they gradually achieved mastery over previously fatal diseases. It is in the field of disease—where the biological cause of an illness is understood—that medicine is most likely to be of value. But identifying new diseases, and developing the corresponding treatments, is tough going. It can be done—the sequencing of the human genome revealed the existence of more than 1,800 disease-causing genes, for example.[3] Nevertheless, constrained by the demand for sound scientific research evidence, with all the expense this entails, identifying genuinely new diseases is a relatively challenging way of adding to the medical encyclopaedia.

Illnesses, on the other hand, are a much more fruitful line of inquiry. A new illness can be created simply by identifying a reasonably large group of people who all report a sufficiently similar cluster of experiences. The tedious requirement to establish the underlying reason why this may be so, or to be confident that the cause is in any way biological, is entirely avoided when working within the freedoms of an illness model. Thus unpleasant experiences that may have as much to do with the individual's personality, their social circumstances or their sense of contractual and political grievance, or which are simply the zeitgeist of the day, are readily transformed into illnesses.

This differentiation between illness and disease is crucial to an appreciation of why medicalisation is often unhelpful. New illnesses can be spawned at a rate of knots if we don't first require any evidence of biological malfunction before accepting them, yet it is precisely in these circumstances that an effective cure is

THE LAND OF THE BLIND

unlikely to exist. The historian Edward Shorter has written about how a society's conception of illness is constantly evolving, and the role of the doctor in signalling to the community whether the individual's constellation of symptoms constitutes a valid illness. If it does, this transforms the person into a patient, with all the attendant ramifications, both social and medical.[ii] When the individual and societal benefits of this process outweigh the harms, we can say that the new illness has utility.

Possible benefits, for example, might include greater awareness and recognition of illnesses generated by environmental factors such as new technology, or a more adapted and helpful understanding of 'old' illnesses.[iii] As medical technology advances, it is sometimes possible to elucidate an underlying disease process that is causative for the illness. For instance, psychological and neurological concepts are increasingly being harmoniously synthesised in the field of neuropsychiatry, as the biomedical basis of previously purely psychiatric disorders such as schizophrenia becomes better understood. Thus illness recognition can be an important first step toward focussing disease research, in the manner of Sydenham.

Drawbacks might include the wastage of expensive medical resource—if the new illness is a problem overwhelmingly amenable to behavioural change on the part of the individual, or wider social change, rather than medical treatment—or social

---

[ii] In *From Paralysis to Fatigue*, Shorter expounds the theory that at any given time in society there is an array of symptoms that are recognised as acceptable and legitimate (the 'symptom pool'), and that changes in attitude and scientific understanding drives a turnover of this pool, with some symptoms departing and new ones appearing.

[iii] For example, the much better neuroscientific insights into post-traumatic stress disorder as compared with the crude conception of 'shell-shock' or neurasthenia.

division, if the medicalisation of certain negative aspects of human behaviour complicates the resolution of disputes and creates a sense of unfairness.[iv] Whilst there is utility to many new illnesses, history equally provides plenty of examples where the concept of illness was stretched beyond absurdity. These tend to reveal something about the moral and political mores of the period, and the foolishness of doctors.

Onania: or, the heinous sin of self-pollution was authored anonymously in 1724.[4] For the next 150 years, Victorian physicians remained comedically obsessed with the frightful physical and psychological consequences of masturbation. In 1865 Dr Henry Maudsley, benefactor of what is now the UK's most prestigious psychiatric hospital, lectured that those who had not been able to desist from interfering with themselves were suffering 'a serious mental disease', and a fatal one at that: 'the sooner he sinks to his degraded rest, the better for himself, and the better for the world, which is well rid of him.'[5] When different sexualities and gender identities were viewed as depravities, they were routinely categorised as mental disorders. The worldwide reference source for mental health conditions categorised homosexuality as a mental disorder until 1973, downgraded it to 'sexual orientation disturbance' thereafter, and only completely removed it from the manual in 1987—a rare instance of an illness departing its mortal coil, only to be replaced by myriad other new 'afflictions' more in keeping with the times.[6]

In 1851 the American physician Samuel Cartwright described drapetomania, the supposedly curious tendency for slaves to become obsessed with making attempts to flee for their freedom.

[iv] This is arguably true, for example, of the tendency to classify negative and undesirable behavioural patterns as personality disorders (where it is generally recognised that the effectiveness of medical treatment is quite limited).

This was inexplicable in the eyes of many slave-owners at the time, given their interpretation of what the Bible had ordained as the natural state of affairs, so mental illness was invoked as the only possible cause of such behaviour. Cartwright postulated that the problem was masters who 'made themselves too familiar with [their slaves], treating them as equals', and proposed that a parental mixture of kindness and discipline was the remedy: 'They have only to be kept in that state and treated like children ... to prevent and cure them from running away.'[7] A balanced telling of the tale requires note that Cartwright's thesis was quickly pilloried in the enlightened northern states, a satirical editorial appearing in the *Buffalo Medical Journal* a few years later.[8]

A partial understanding of science can generate illness too. As science and technology advance, and populations become scared of environmental factors of which they were previously unaware—speed, vibration, ionising radiation, electromagnetic radiation, chemicals—so there is the potential for the quacks to scaremonger. In the right dose and in the right circumstances, each of these phenomena has the potential to harm human health, but their propensity to do so is vastly overstated by the generations that are first to become aware of them. Thus the Victorian preoccupation that the unaccustomed speed and jolting movements of the new steam trains were causing an epidemic of 'railway spine'.

Our more modern fixations include the compulsive statistical analysis of leukaemia incidence rates in the vicinity of nuclear power plants, in a determination to find a direct causal link that does not exist;[9] electromagnetic hypersensitivity syndrome, which has already attracted compensation in the UK despite not being officially recognised as a condition;[10] and multiple chemical sensitivity (MCS) syndrome. At the outset of the new millennium in Nova Scotia, a ban came into force on wearing scented products—including deodorants, shampoos and perfumes—in indoor public places such as local government buildings, libraries, hospitals, classrooms, courts and public transport vehicles. *The Globe and Mail* dubbed this move to counter the growing menace of MCS 'Non-scents in Nova Scotia'.[11] Later in the '00s, public bodies in places such as Minnesota, Maryland and Portland, Oregon followed suit. At first a concern peculiar to North America, that hot-house for medicalisation, similar anxieties concerning MCS have begun to metastasise across the Atlantic.[12]

Conditions are born and achieve recognition through their inclusion in diagnostic compendia. There are two in widespread use. These are the World Health Organization's *International Classification of Diseases* (ICD), currently in its eleventh iteration and known as ICD-11, and the American Psychiatric Association's *Diagnostic and Statistical Manual of Mental Disorders*, in its fifth variant (DSM-V).[13] The convention for cases of mental illness is to use DSM-V.

When DSM-V was published in 2013, it attracted a great deal of controversy. Traditionally there has been something of a battle between what we could call the British school, which holds that devising new conditions is a process that needs to be undertaken carefully and cautiously, and its more enthusiastic American counterpart. DSM-V, an American creation, predictably included various new conditions that some might consider to be evidence of our ongoing desire to push the bounds of medicine and common sense. Equally, it watered down the diagnostic criteria for a number of conditions already in existence. Controversial new disorders included Caffeine Withdrawal, Cannabis Withdrawal, Hoarding, and Disruptive Mood Dysregulation Disorder.[v]

---

[v] A disorder of children characterised by 'severe and recurrent temper outbursts that are grossly out of proportion in intensity or duration to the situation. These occur, on average, three or more times each week for one

Disorders for which the diagnostic threshold has been lowered include Post-Traumatic Stress Disorder, which can now be acquired vicariously if trauma has befallen a close friend or family member, and the worrisomely titled 'Intermittent Explosive Disorder'. This can be diagnosed in children as young as six and is characterised by 'recurrent outbursts that demonstrate an inability to control impulses'.[vi] As proof that satire is not dead, hypochondriasis was removed from DSM-V, as a word deemed to have pejorative connotations.

In addition to being an exhaustive catalogue of kosher illnesses, DSM-V includes 'Section III', which gives advance notice of new conditions that are in the shortlist for entry into DSM-VI, but for which society needs some further softening up first. This is the purgatory where afflictions such as Caffeine Use Disorder and Internet Gaming Disorder—a dead cert since it has already been included in ICD-11[14]—patiently await their beatification in the next edition. The American Psychiatric Association describes Section III as something that 'should be of equal importance to clinicians, because there they will find diagnostic tools that can be used today and also anticipate an evolving understanding of psychiatric illness tomorrow.'[15] It is aimed at the kind of people who would wait overnight to be at the front of the queue for the latest iPhone; the early-adopting pioneers of medicalisation who are seeking patients as the unwitting beta-testers for their preferred whimsy.

---

year or more.' The condition is very different, the APA assures us, from temper tantrums.

[vi] More specifically, verbal or physical aggression (not leading to damage to property or physical injury) that occurs at least twice a week for at least 3 months, or 3 outbursts involving injury or 'destruction' within a 1-year period. IED is an acronym that has unfortunate connotations these days; this diagnosis literally makes little terrors out of children.

In tribunals and courtrooms, ICD-11 and DSM-V are treated with the gravity of sacred texts by those who are naive about how ridiculous and subjective the distinction between what is or is not a pukka illness. Lawyers have a compulsion to establish whether something is a 'recognised' medical condition. In reality, the type of illnesses prevalent in a society, and listed in these tomes, reveal as much about its culture, attitudes and beliefs as they do about its biology. A society's conceptions of illness are a mirror to that society itself: its follies, prejudices and hobby-horses as much as its scientific prowess.

Fifty or sixty years ago, medical practitioners worked largely within a disease-based model. Accepting claims of illness from those with no discernible disease was the exception rather than the norm. The advantage of this approach was that it equipped the doctor with the power to normalise the patient's experience for them. In this way the plight of people with cancer, heart disease, neurological impairment, terminal illness and severe psychiatric illness such as schizophrenia or bipolar affective disorder would be differentiated from those with heavy flu, a touch of backache, anxiety about their upcoming exams, or distress at the treatment they had received from their manager. The evolution in society's attitude towards illness that has occurred since—the rise of 'stress' being a particularly egregious example—has been reflected in the changing nature of the conditions cited as a reason for claiming sickness benefits. The proportion of claimants claiming sickness benefits for a mental health problem more than doubled from 21.4 per cent in 1995 to 46.5 per cent by 2014.[16] For those in work, stress-related illnesses accounted for nigh-on half of all working days lost to ill health in 2016–17.[17]

When this ostensibly dramatic increase in mental illness is discussed, the question is inevitably asked: 'Is it real?' Is the sum of collective human psychopathology now genuinely higher than 150 years ago, when the infant mortality rate was approximately one in seven, most people were dead by their early forties, and lives were spent working in Dickensian conditions?[18] Or a century ago, when families throughout the country mourned the deaths of a million young men and had to cope with the return of almost 2 million more who had been maimed, many gruesomely?[19] Or, rather, is the rise an illusory one—the explanation not being that people are more ill, but that we diagnose illness more readily?

Arguments can be made either way. As the statistics above illustrate, there can be little doubt that in many ways life was much harder just a few generations ago. If mental illness was genuinely a rarer entity in those days, then this would provide strong empirical evidence to support Illich's theory that our predecessors' belief systems were of more help to them in enduring physical and emotional hardship than ours are to us. Alternatively, some argue that twenty-first-century life poses entirely novel and insidious threats to our mental health. Amongst the commonly identified potential culprits are the demise of traditional family structures, the monotony of industrial jobs, the precariousness of zero-hours contracts in the services sector, social media, the 24-hour news cycle and permanent connection of the digital age, and the decline of religion in a technological age.

The atomisation of the traditional extended family was achieved through the combination of birth control (which reduced the size of families) and greater freedom of travel (which pulled them geographically further apart). Familial support networks are now smaller and more tenuous. There are fewer hands to help when the inevitable crises of life—births, diseases, divorces, bankruptcies and deaths—intercede. Industrialisation has in some ways degraded us and our experience of life. In *Zen and the Art of Motorcycle Maintenance*, Robert Pirsig explored how—for many people—having some sense of purpose, seeing a tangible result for their endeavours, can be so important. Yet since Henry Ford ushered in the era of mass production, a high proportion of the workforce has found itself in mundane, seemingly pointless and ultimately soul-sapping jobs. Workers are forever assembling one nondescript component with another as the conveyor ceaselessly rolls on, never getting to enjoy the thrill and satisfaction of seeing the culmination of the manufacturing process. Most of us have at least a streak of the completer-finisher in us.

In 1920s America, the craze of flagpole-sitting captured the public imagination. Individuals seeking publicity and egged on by friends would see how long they could sit aloft a flagpole as a feat of endurance. In 1924 Alvin 'Shipwreck' Kelly, who popularised the hobby, achieved a time of thirteen hours and thirteen minutes. This was bettered by various other enthusiasts in subsequent years before he reclaimed his title in 1930s with a record of forty-nine days. Flagpole-sitting itself was an uncomfortable, absurd and pointless exercise, but for a while it was a means of achieving recognition and prize money.[vii] Popular culture has used it as a clever metaphor for how many people feel about their dystopian modern lives.[viii] A career of thirty years spent on a mass production line makes even less sense than thirty days atop a flagpole, in terms of our desire for a life well lived.

Many of these traditional, manufacturing jobs have been displaced to the Far East as a result of global market forces. The same allegation of mind-numbing repetitiveness can be levelled against many of the service-sector roles in call centres and fast

---

[vii] Until the Great Depression of 1929, after which its popularity waned, as people had no time for such fripperies.

[viii] The '90s indie rock band Harvey Danger captured the dysthymic malaise of modern living especially well in the lyrics of *Flagpole Sitta:* 'I'm not sick but I'm not well/And I'm so hot 'cause I'm in hell/I'm not sick but I'm not well/And it's a sin to live so well.'

food emporia that have replaced them. Worse, if work histori-cally was boring, but at least predictable and secure, many mod-ern service-sector roles in the 'gig economy' achieve the toxic blend of being both mindless and precariousness in nature. The emergence of zero-hours contracts in sectors such as taxi driving, fast food delivery, couriering and hospitality seem liable to pose new and insidious threats to mental health.

Humans are social creatures, and how we feel we compare with our peers is highly deterministic of how we feel about ourselves. Hence, social media is now widely perceived as the great evil of our age. With the relentless stream of images from smug attention-seekers enjoying—or rather, appearing to enjoy—lifestyles of ease and happiness, our sense of our own inadequacy is endlessly rein-forced. The argument that social media grossly distorts our frame of reference is a plausible one. Worse, many seem to find it hard to contemplate being prised away from the devices channelling such bilge to them, along with the other incessant streams of intrigue, gossip and 'fake news'. Fear Of Missing Out leads us to choose such ephemeral trivia, displayed with an insomnia-inducing glow on our tablet and phone screens, over the refreshing sleep needed for good mental health. The ubiquitous uptake of such technology within such a short space of time, and its dramatic disruptions to our social life and diurnal rhythms, represent a vast—yet largely unquestioned—social experiment. In time, we may come to view it as being no less harmful than the unregulated introduction of a new addictive drug.

These are all factors with which our predecessors did not have to contend, and which seem to be making us ill. There is even the theory that—in the absence of having to worry about the prime-val needs of survival and sustenance—our ape brains are instead forced to occupy themselves by ruminating incessantly over more thorny, existential desires that are that much harder to satisfy. This requires a little explanation. The great majority of life that has ever existed on Earth has been in the guise of more primitive organisms, which, even if they might have been conscious, were not curious or self-aware to an extent that they might contemplate what would happen next week, what might be over the next hill, or what the point of the universe might be. They were gene-carrying automatons. In accordance with the evolutionary principles described by Darwin, and latterly Dawkins, these ancestors were perfected to endure long enough to reproduce as plentifully as possible—and nothing more. They passed from dust and back to it in an endless series of life cycles, on the planet and interacting with it, yet oblivious to their own existence.

Selection pressures acted on these biological droids such that they developed progressively more powerful on-board computers, able to remember, plan, think in abstract terms and critically appraise choices. In other words, to worry. From an evolutionary standpoint, worry confers a survival advantage. By repeatedly imagining how a sequence of events might unfold in the future, we give ourselves the chance to prepare and to perform better. For example, by fretting about our demise if we don't procure water or berries in a sufficiently timely way, and thinking about the strategies we have used in the past for finding them, we give ourselves the opportunity to prepare and plan for the next day's foraging, so that the chances of it being successful are as high as possible. Being entirely carefree might theoretically be pleasant for self-aware organisms, but it is not a trait likely to endure in the gene-pool for very long.

It seems likely, then, that we are hardwired to worry, and that our worries are largely kept in check by securing the things we worry about. The cumulative power of billions of human brains over time has generated technology that has made worries about shelter and sustenance a thing of the past for most people in developed countries. It may be that our instinctual need to worry means that we now merely fixate on different things. And it may be our

THE LAND OF THE BLIND

downfall that these more rarefied worries are intrinsically more difficult to soothe: how are we here, what is our purpose, what does it all mean? This is the unanswerable existential angst of any sapient set of atoms able to contemplate its own existence.[ix]

Human consciousness is the ultimate biological capability, as evidenced by the ubiquity and dominance of humankind since its emergence. But this supreme computer was a byproduct of an evolutionary arms race, constructed not by design but by Dawkins' Blind Watchmaker. Its processing power was helpful in solving the more practical problems of day-to-day life, such as where to find food and how to kill it, but its operating system posed entirely new existential challenges for organisms that became conscious. As creatures we became capable of torturing ourselves by posing unknowable questions. The human neocortex—the most recent part of the brain in evolutionary terms, and the most sophisticated—is indeed a double-edged sword.

This would constitute what we might call a kind of Maslowian neurosis. With his hierarchy of needs theory, Maslow suggested in the mid-twentieth century that there was a series of incremental needs in our life, waypoints on our journey to what he called our self-actualisation.[x] These ranged from the most basic physical needs to the immaterial need of finding purpose in our

---

[ix] In his book *Cosmos*, the astrophysicist Carl Sagan describes our cosmic self-awareness by saying, 'We have begun to contemplate our origins: starstuff pondering the stars; organized assemblages of ten billion billion billion atoms considering the evolution of atoms; tracing the long journey by which, here at least, consciousness arose.' The suggestion that this is a unique awareness in the cosmos is a hypothesis yet to be disproved, but may be in the future if alien life is found, at which time the comparison of intergalactic approaches to psychotherapy will make an interesting study.

[x] Maslow expounded this theory in his 1943 paper 'A Theory of Human Motivation', published in the journal *Psychological Review*.

life. We can imagine a corresponding set of escalating worries. In earlier phases of civilisation, few people could ever truly escape the concerns of the physical world and we could reason that their worries, whilst intense, might have been simpler to placate. Whilst modern life may have freed many people from concerns about their physical world, it might also mean that their brains—hardwired to worry and with plenty of spare processor capacity—are now free to generate metaphysical angst instead.

We are what we always have been, since we were the first primitive bacteria: vehicles for genes engaged in a ceaseless quest to survive and replicate. The novel twist is that 'we'—in the form of conscious neocortices—are now spectators to the struggle, 3 pounds of gelatinous electrochemistry encased in a bony skull with audiovisual inputs from the outside world. We have become passengers along for this ride spanning from birth through mating to death, distracting ourselves en route with interminable questions to which there can be no answer. In this analysis, belief is conceived as an innate human need: tried-and-tested religious and cultural belief systems evolved over hundreds and thousands of years, memes that propagated only if they were capable of soothing our existential angst to a bearable level, and which were therefore pleasant for us. Without these ointments, humans seem uniquely vulnerable in the animal kingdom. The explosion of science and technology in the post-Enlightenment period, so quickly supplanting so many of these carefully nurtured belief systems, may have denuded us of our metaphysical skin.

After the 1969 moon landing of the Apollo XI mission, the BBC broadcast a live edition of its current affairs programme *Panorama*. It was astutely titled 'The Impact on Earth', at a time when all eyes were cast upward into the stars. Luminaries on the studio panel included the science fiction writer Brian Aldiss and the historian Hugh Trevor-Roper. When the episode aired, the returning spacemen had yet to shake the moon dust from their suits back on the home planet; they were just embarking on their 238,855-mile journey back to Earth from the Sea of Tranquillity. In retrospect it is fascinating how quickly wise minds began urging caution amidst the euphoria at this milestone, characterised by Brian Aldiss as the realisation of a million-year-old ambition of the neocortex. He expressed the fear that technology 'will become enthroned as the new religion, and that it may well be taking over now ... This tremendous triumph of technology may merely lead to a thirst for more technology'. As Illich would write soon after, although in classical rather than gastronomic terms, technology might be to the proverbial takeaway what traditional belief systems are to a homemade meal: short-term satisfaction, but a poor substitute for the more filling fare of freshly made meat with two vegetables. Technology is a distracting spectacle, but only temporarily. It is not one that is an effective long-term palliative for our nagging questions and doubts.

Trevor-Roper in turn observed a danger of the technological age: that people might be enslaved by this thirst, which would never quite be quenched—that the real battle would be to 'maintain people's humanity, to stop people becoming robots ... It's always possible that great technological changes will enslave people.' When asked to forecast what the next fifty years might bring—meaning by the year 2019—he answered that he could not, and that what was needed was 'perpetual vigilance'.[20] Indeed, now that those fifty years have passed, an ever-higher proportion of people in developed countries report unhappiness with their lives, and feeling trapped in the jobs they need to undertake in order to generate the income needed to consume ever more technology. It is difficult to escape the conclusion that many are caught in consumerism and have indeed been enslaved. Collectively, they have been unable to develop any new and more adapted belief system—something beyond traditional religion but nevertheless immaterial and addressing existential angst and achieving self-actualisation in a way that being a consumer of technology cannot. Trevor-Roper, were he alive, might conclude that we have not been vigilant enough.

We can postulate various reasons, then, as to why the rise in rates of mental illness might be real. But the hypothesis cannot be tested, because measuring mental health in a sufficiently objective way for comparisons to be made between one generation and the next is impossible. In statistical and scientific terms, the attempts of ICD-11 or DSM-V to try and quantify the proportion of people with a mental health problem are as arbitrary as trying to assert what proportion of people are grumpy or cheerful. Commentators play fast and loose with the numbers they bandy around. The most commonly parroted factoid is that one in four people will experience a mental health problem in their lifetime. Yet, when researchers questioned those citing this statistic about its provenance, the responses proved to be hazy. They concluded that it was likely appealing as a Goldilocks number: high enough to have dramatic impact and be in tune with campaigns to destigmatise the issue, but low enough to remain credible.[21]

The field of mental health has an inflation rate to rival that of the Weimar Republic. In a 'myths and facts' section, the website of the charitable campaign Time to Change reports as 'fact'—thankfully not as clichéd 'scientific fact', though that is clearly the insinuation—that 'Around 1 in 4 people will experience a mental health problem this year'.[22] Not to be outdone, the Mind website tells us that 'In England, 1 in 6 people report experiencing a common mental health problem (such as anxiety and depression) in any given week'.[23] These are simply not figures that can be trusted in the same way that we can be reasonably confident, for example, about the number of patients who have had heart attacks, have had legs amputated, or have died. The latter are what clinicians refer to as hard end-points: there is little room for ambiguity. Reports of mental illness, on the other hand, are what they are: opinions dependent in the final analysis on where we arbitrarily choose to draw the line between normality and illness.

One of the challenges of tracking trends in mental illness is the relative lack of hard end-points, whereas these are more commonplace in physical medicine: rates of stroke, heart attack, amputation, death and so on. Suicide rates are the closest thing to a hard end-point in the field of psychiatry. They are not a perfect proxy measure for psychiatric ill health for many reasons, not least because some people who kill themselves are not mentally ill,[xi] but they can at least be measured fairly precisely.

[xi] This difficult and thought-provoking observation is made as an aside in the opening remarks of a chapter entitled 'Dicing With Death' in Andrew Malleson's *The Medical Runaround*. Its casual introduction is clearly intended to alert the reader that, if they have assumed that intention to kill oneself is synonymous with mental illness, this may need some deeper contemplation. The Sanati article that is referenced offers a good discussion of the challenging issues that arise, not least the concepts that—in extreme circumstances—suicide may be a rational option, and that our revulsion to this may reveal more about our own fears (especially, amongst healthcare workers, of being blamed for acquiescence) than about the existence of a powerful, absolute, philosophical or ethical argument to the contrary. The antithesis would, for example, require us to deny Socrates his reason, or concentration camp inmates their last remaining freedom to choose. If these seem esoteric points of reference, Sanati cites the examples of Debbie Purdy and Daniel James as more relatable examples. Cases of severely ill people, or people in otherwise intolerable circumstances, who feel—quite lucidly—that death is preferable to their existence, are perhaps more common than we care to think. *London Journal of Primary Care* (2009) 2(2): 93094. Does suicide always indicate a mental illness? A Sanati. Available at https://www.ncbi.nlm.nih.gov/pmc/articles/PMC4222167/ [Accessed 6 October 2018].

Whilst the Western media is rightly concerned about the tragedy of suicide and the issue receives a great deal of press, it would be a mistake to think that suicide is a new phenomenon or even one that is on the rise. Quite the contrary: the suicide rate has been in decline for most of the last few decades, falling by approximately a quarter between 1981 and 2016.[24] This is even accounting for a lesser, upward tick in the years that followed the 2008 financial crisis, a rise that peaked in 2013 at a level still substantially lower than the rates seen after the recessions of the 1980s and '90s.[25] Men aged over seventy-five were more likely in the 1980s to commit suicide than any other demographic, and the suicide rate in this group more than halved during the same quarter-century period (1981–2016).[26] In the years since the financial crisis, this long-term reduction in the suicide rate has resumed; the fall in the suicide rate between 2015 and 2016 was the steepest recorded for more than twenty years.[27] What data there is, relating to this hardest of hard end-points, does not sit neatly with the hypothesis that rates of serious mental illness are on the rise.

Given the subjective nature of the process of making a mental illness diagnosis, there can be no definitive answer to the question of whether the rise in mental illness is real or artificial, only hypotheses. Mental health problems simply cannot be conceptualised in the same way as physical diseases such as coronary artery disease or multiple sclerosis. Errors in public policy will ensue if we seek to pretend otherwise. Yet the politically correct trope that mental health problems should always be assumed to have an equivalence with physical health problems has been enshrined within the Health and Social Care Act (2012), the NHS Constitution and the NHS Mandate, creating an obligation on the NHS to deliver 'parity of esteem' between physical and mental health.[28] With time this approach may prove to be too simplistic, and one we come to regret.

The government's 2017 report *Thriving at Work* contains another dubious mental health statistic: this time, the claim that

300,000 people—or 0.93 per cent of the working population[xii]—lose their jobs each year as the result of a long-term mental health condition (LTMHC).[29] The researchers derived this statistic using data from the two-wave longitudinal Labour Force Survey,[xiii] which asks respondents a series of questions about their health and their employment status on two occasions, three months apart. The statisticians compared how many people self-reported having both a job and a LTMHC on the first occasion with those who did not have a job but still had a LTMHC on the second. From this they calculated the percentage of people with a LTMHC who had fallen out of work and, by extrapolating the data from this sample to the UK working population as a whole, arrived at the 300,000 figure.

There are profound problems with this statistic. Whether or not respondents were deemed to have a mental health problem depended solely on whether or not they considered themselves to have one; no objectivity was applied. And to talk emotively about people 'losing their jobs' implies that these are people who are dismissed, as it would be a strange way to describe a situation where someone resigns from their employment. But when the researchers were making their calculation they did not distinguish between people who were dismissed against their wishes, those who were glad to be dismissed,[xiv] those who resigned, and those who lost their jobs for reasons entirely unrelated to their health such as redundancy. This was despite the fact that the

---

[xxii] Assuming a working population of 32.1m, as per ONS data (the UK Labour Market Statistical Bulletin for October 2017).

[xxiii] Specifically, four sets of data (Q2 of 2016 to Q2 of 2017) from the Labour Force Survey (LFS) longitudinal datasets of the Office for National Statistics.

[xiv] Some employees prefer dismissal to resignation as it may facilitate their access to out-of-work benefits, or to redundancy pay.

dataset the researchers used did include more granular data about the reasons for leaving employment: respondents were given eleven reasons to choose from.

Even the authors heavily caveat their work and acknowledge the figure may be an overestimate. But we are back to the problem of dubious statistics being used to argue the case for a mental health pandemic. How many of those deemed to have a LTMHC did not have a serious psychiatric problem at all, but were experiencing chronic unhappiness with their job? For them, leaving that employment may have been the best thing that could have happened to them. The report infers that their departure was enforced upon them, yet some will have left—entirely appropriately—through resignation, and of those who were dismissed, there is no way of knowing what proportion were pleased by the action of their employer.

The etymology of the term 'mental illness' is clearly complex, but do the intergenerational differences in what we consider 'normal' have any bearing on how we should approach the problem of sickness? It doesn't really matter whether the sky is falling and there are now masses of mentally disturbed people, or whether we simply diagnose mental illness more readily. In either case, medicine and psychiatry cannot hope to solve the problem, because their resources are finite. Reason must prevail. Resources must not be squandered on those who, in relative terms, are well; and all but the most sick need to continue working, at least if we wish to keep the lights on and the national infrastructure running.

If modern life is relatively benign in a historical context, and we are medicalising excessively so that people with common physical and emotional problems are being classed as ill, then it follows that—in a clinical assessment of the trade-off between risks and benefits—most people should remain untreated, and certainly not prescribed psychoactive drugs. It is therefore concerning that the rise in prescriptions for antidepressants is steeper than for any other category of drug. The number of anti-depressant prescriptions in 2016 was more than double that of just a decade earlier.[30] We might think that doctors would be especially mindful of the dangers of prescribing to pregnant women, as there are two human lives to think about and, in most cases, the mother will be as concerned for the baby's health as for their own. These medicines cross the placenta and the foetal blood-brain barrier to reach the foetal brain. The prescribing behaviour of doctors, when it comes to pregnant women, is therefore an interesting place to look if we are fearful that doctors are prescribing with reckless abandon.

One study found that, in 2004–10, 3.7 per cent of pregnant women in England, Scotland and Northern Ireland—and 4.5 per cent in Wales—were prescribed antidepressants.[31] As ever, the Americans blaze the trail; a study of over 1 million pregnancies amongst women enrolled in the Medicaid programme between 2000 and 2007 found that 8.1 per cent were prescribed an antidepressant during pregnancy.[32] This is decade-old data; the current rate is likely to be frighteningly high, given that antidepressant prescription rates generally have doubled in the intervening period.[33] The current practice of doling out industrial quantities of antidepressants—and especially dousing the brains of developing babies in psychoactive drugs by prescribing them to their mothers—may one day prove to be a further entry in the lengthening catalogue of harms caused by doctors who are too trigger-happy with their prescription pads. There is early tentative evidence that these babies may be at increased risk of, amongst other things, autism and psychiatric disorders.[34]

Even if modern life truly is making people sick to this extent, and the scale of medical treatment of mental health problems is anywhere near justified, then plainly we should not be relying on medicine to resuscitate its victims. Instead it is modern life that needs to change. Addressing our present dystopia is not a matter of industrial-scale medical or psychotherapeutic manipulation of minds. When casualty departments were inundated as motoring became accessible to the masses, because no-one had yet thought to devise safety measures such as seatbelts and anti-lock brakes, the solution was to design better cars—not to build more hospitals.

In fact, what happens if a populace is placated into thinking of their plight as a medical problem rather than one of cultural malaise or poor social and political governance? The political mechanisms that address important issues of social justice may be subverted. Everybody may be distracted and looking in the wrong place for a solution. The stress epidemic is the apotheosis of this,[xv] a medical outburst of the recurring tensions in labour relations which once—in an age of collectivism—would instead have manifested themselves in strike action. These tensions are still a challenge to the social and political system, but perhaps more honestly stated.

Ours is a grotesquely medicalised society. Until the advent of modern medicine, we relied on cultural or religious belief systems to cope with the uncomfortable experiences of our being—with our symptoms.[xvi] Illich observed how the different role models of major world religions—the thinker, the martyr, the warrior—provided templates that assisted the individual in making some sense of their predicament and teaching them how they should endure it. Importantly, these were belief systems that did not deny the harsh realities of peoples' lives but instead convinced them that they could survive them. They did not promise

---

[xv] The HSE has calculated that work-related stress, work-related depression or work-related anxiety was the cause for 49% of all working days lost to ill health in 2016/17 (*Work-related Stress, Depression or Anxiety Statistics in Great Britain 2017*).

[xvi] Symptom is derived from the Greek word meaning misfortune.

believers that suffering could be avoided, but taught that there was a purpose to it, which itself provided a means of coping.

The yin and yang of our existence were first described by Chinese philosophers around 5,000 years ago. The idea that all suffering constitutes a problem we can or should seek to fix is an error of thinking, a hubris. It is an alluring fallacy that appears plausible to modern eyes because, since Sydenham and the Enlightenment, medical technology seems to have performed miracles. Most Westerners have excessive confidence in medicine, inculcated subliminally in them from birth (see Chapter 5). They have greater scholastic exposure to the work of Christian Barnard, Edward Jenner and Alexander Fleming than to Confucius. Their assumption is that we can combat the ethereal foes of loss, sadness and angst as assuredly as we can the tangible ones of failing organs and microbes. They fail to appreciate the limits to medicine, the term Illich used as the title for his seminal book—its relative impotence when applied to those illnesses that we have defined although they exist outside of a disease model.

In assuming this supremacy as the solace in our lives, medicine has estranged us from the cultural and religious coping mechanisms that were available to our predecessors. The individual is disempowered. The effect of this is that we become deskilled in our ability to cope with reality, which is frequently adverse.[xvii] Regaining our capacity to cope with life in the twenty-first century will be a matter of social and political

xvii What Illich termed 'social and cultural iatrogenesis', iatrogenesis referring to the harm inadvertently caused by medicine's attempts to heal. The dangers of drug side-effects, or inappropriate surgical violence (such as denuding generations of children of their tonsils or lobotomising disturbed people), are obvious. Individual disempowerment, and growing dependency on medicine, are more subtle—and all the more pernicious for it.

upheaval, not in the superficial sense of class war, but more pro-foundly, through the development of belief systems in keeping with the age. These cannot involve a return to the same religions as served us in the prescientific age; but nor can they be dehu-manising in the way that our current worship of technology has proved to be. Until we find the answer, the ingredients for endemic levels of sickness are all there. A medicalised populace will naturally seek succour from its doctor priests, who—as we know—have both poorly effective treatments and a readiness to certify sickness.

Ultimately we need a disciplined, continent approach to the diagnosis of mental illness. Nowadays, naively and simplistically, we think of mental illness as disturbances of an individual's thoughts, feelings or behaviours that distress them (or others), or which impair them in the conduct of their lives. In and of itself, this is an open-ended definition, and in theory everyone could be ill. This is a state we seem to be fast approaching, given the statistics relating to antidepressant usage. We have forgotten the second crucial aspect to any concept of mental illness, which is that the distress or impairment needs to be to an abnormal extent.[xviii] In other words, mental illness is defined relative to the prevailing norms within any given culture at any given time. It is this additional criterion that imposes sensible limits to illness. It is a caveat that the acolytes of the psychiatric movement have

[xviii] In its 'Key Facts' section about mental disorders, the World Health Organization describes them as 'characterized by a combination of abnor-mal thoughts, perceptions, emotions, behaviour and relationships with others'. Few contemplate sufficiently carefully the significance of the word 'abnormal': it is a normative construct, rather than one that is value-laden. In a hypothetical society where more than 50 per cent of the population were on antidepressants, it would be those who were not medicated who would have to be classed as abnormal.

overlooked in their arrogance and their eagerness to impose their often self-interested 'solutions' on society. The medical model has justifiably attracted vehement criticism from many quarters as a simplistic and dehumanising way of conceptualising physical disability, with pleas for a more holistic, social approach to the issue. Yet the progressive intrusion of the medical model into the arena of mental health, and the labelling of progressively more people as having mental health problems—without regard to social aspects—seems to pass largely unchallenged.

The arguments could run and run as to whether there is genuinely more mental illness these days, or whether life is tougher or we are weaker—but they have as much practical relevance as debating how many angels can dance on the head of a pin. Either way, we should reserve the valuable resources of our finite healthcare system for treating the sickest people. That means thinking about the problem from a supply-side perspective as much as from one of demand.

Sickness is relative: everyone has their problems, but most people need to be working to support those who simply cannot. In the land of the blind, the one-eyed man is king. For everyone's sake, he cannot be allowed to indulge himself indefinitely in his monocular grief to the extent that he must be signed off. At some point he needs to stop bothering his counsellor and his ophthalmologist, and get back to work: for there are blind people who rely on him doing so.

11

FANNING THE FLAMES

Medicalisation bestows doctors with the power to create sickness in two ways.

First, by giving them an aura of omnipotence, society then feels confident entrusting them with certification. In a medicalised society, laypeople are raised on a diet of documentaries and 'breakthrough' news stories about the success of medicine in treating diseases. Credulous belief in the medical model empowers the Western doctor in the same way that belief in spirits gives legitimacy to the shaman. The subsequent requirement for doctors to collude in the disreputable practice of certification, helping absentees to feel vindicated in their decision to stay home from work, is the most obvious way in which medical practitioners empty workplaces up and down the country and boost the ratings for daytime television programmes. Through the pretence that the doctor is able to make an objective assessment, people who would be capable of work—given the right support and encouragement from those around them—in practice go sick, if their request for a certificate is granted. The great majority of the time, that is what will happen.[1]

But medicalisation also provides a second, more creative, way in which doctors cause sickness. As well as giving them the power to legitimise sickness, we have also entrusted them with the authority to adjudicate on what constitutes a medical condition in the first place. As examples such as onania, drapetomania, and intermittent explosive disorder show, there has been and remains a common sense deficit amongst the medical profession which means that our trust in them to define the sensible limits to their own services is probably misplaced. Through rampant medicalisation—transforming the way that society views a particular problem, such that it comes to be seen as one with a medical basis and a solution in medicine—doctors devise exciting new illnesses which can then generate further sick-notes. In other words, medicalisation creates new opportunities for sickness to manifest itself. If the cornucopia of human illness is thought of as a coal mine, medicalisation occurs when aspiring absentees and their doctors strike into entirely new and as yet untapped seams of coal.

To address the problem of sickness, then, we need to address the problem of medicalisation. How do you demedicalise a hopelessly medicalised society? Well, the first maxim of public health is that prevention is better than cure. This is a good rule of thumb when planning how best to reduce the incidence of cervical cancer, or dental caries, or rickets. The mass immunisation of children against the human papilloma virus, the fluoridisation of drinking water and the fortification of bread with vitamin D are all sheep-dip approaches to improving health that have the merit of being effective.

Disease prevention also relies heavily on education. Knowledge is power, and knowing how to use a condom or an automated external defibrillator can save your life or that of someone else. But mishaps arise when this prevention/education mantra is transplanted from the disease context in which it originated into one of illness. Campaigns intended to educate people about illness have less predictable results. If those illnesses have a perverse appeal to many people, or are seen as an easy route to compensation, or are the product of mass hysteria or delusional thinking, then attempts to eradicate or at least to manage them by clichéd efforts to 'raise awareness' may be useless or even counterproductive.

In the 2006 television documentary *Stephen Fry: The Secret Life of the Manic Depressive*, the subject of the programme said that he 'loved' having the condition: 'It's tormented me all my life with the deepest of depressions while giving me the energy and creativity that perhaps has made my career.'[2] Following these and other similar media features on celebrities with bipolar, some psychologists and psychiatrists reported seeing a rise in the number of people inappropriately self-diagnosing themselves as having bipolar affective disorder, formerly a serious psychiatric diagnosis and very much the province of psychiatrists. This has been attributed to the connotations of tortured artistic genius that the documentary lent to the disorder.[3]

The Victorian fad of railway spine, the RSI[i] epidemic of the late 1980s (which flared so spectacularly in Australia), and the ongoing scandal of whiplash are examples of conditions where hysteria and the compensable nature of the problem likely played a large part in explaining the impotence of preventative measures.[4] Safer train travel, more comfortable office work and better cars did not put an end to these problems. Instead, the death knell of such phenomena comes when government calls time on those doctors and lawyers busily skimming the fat from con-

---

[i] The term is used advisedly since the condition was a diagnosis of exclusion; this means that its reference to 'injury', implying something demonstrable, was a misnomer.

fected compensation claims, by imposing limits on the awards that can be made. In 2017 the Ministry of Justice announced such measures for whiplash claims. This was in response to a 50 per cent increase over a decade in the number of road traffic accident-related personal injury claims—90 per cent of which are for whiplash—despite improvements in vehicle design that would have been expected to achieve a reduction.[5] Whiplash will hopefully be the next medicolegal epidemic to become history. If so, its eradication will indeed have been achieved through a public information campaign about whiplash, but in the sense of demonisation rather than raising awareness. Perhaps stress will follow it, when we tire of its promotion.

During an earlier outbreak of unprovable illness allegedly associated with injury, on that occasion of industrial back pain, doctors eventually came to realise that—by and large—the more sensible approach was to normalise and reassure people about what is a commonplace experience. In short, to encourage sufferers to get on with things as best they could.[6] At this stage in the evolution of the stress epidemic, it remains heretical to suggest that initiatives serving to medicalise and catastrophise the previously mundane world of industrial relations may be part of the problem as much as they are the cure.

Royal Mail's Corporate Responsibility Report for 2016/17 mentions 'mental health issues' as one of the leading causes of long-term sickness absence,[7] a vague term that can cover a multitude of sins. It goes on to explain—without irony—that over 2,600 of its managers have watched its mental health awareness films, over 400 have attended 'mental health first aid' training courses, and management has collaborated with the unions to develop new stress risk awareness tools, with the stated aim of early identification of stress-related issues. This is seemingly oblivious to the fact that the preceding year's report had already identified mental health as a priority and had implemented similar measures—but that sickness absence had nevertheless increased.[8]

FANNING THE FLAMES

Some organisations are sufficiently large to warrant the creation of 'wellness' sinecures. These human resources or health and safety professionals are specifically tasked with putting out the fire of the stress epidemic. Yet, for the time being, they seem content to continue pouring petrol over it rather than cold water. There is little likelihood of this changing any time soon. These professionals remain guided by theory, rather than by practical experience of the Molotov cocktail 'solutions' that they have implemented so far. Stress consultancy is in demand, but unfortunately not all consultants within these areas of enterprise offer solutions that are particularly evidence-based. Stress is a big problem for employers, yet also one that they poorly understand, and the conditions for an exploitative market are ripe. Demand is high, whilst customers lack confidence in their ability to appraise the value of the services that they are buying amidst all the psychobabble. The evidence for this is empirical. The scale of the stress problem grows in proportion to the number of academic, lifestyle and wellness experts purporting to have the solution to it, with their stream of papers, blogs and tweets. A confused marketplace remains under the spell of its Svengalis.

Employers can scarcely be criticised for not having devised any informed or sophisticated response to the problem of medicalisation when the same is true of our academic and political leaders and institutions. Confusion reigns at the highest levels of the establishment. Pronouncements about how to tackle the epidemic of mental illness[ii] and the associated strains on mental health services consist exclusively of tired clichés. There are claims that these are stigmatised conditions, and promises to divert more resources to this purportedly under-recognised problem.

[ii] The World Health Organization's 'Depression' fact-sheet describes it as the leading worldwide cause of disability.

In 2016 the government announced a radical transformation of mental health services, in response to the report of an 'independent taskforce'.[9] This taskforce was chaired by Paul Farmer, chief executive of Mind, a mental health charity whose stated purpose is to raise awareness of and improve services for mental illness. The government response to the report was to pledge an additional £1 billion to this end over the following five years.[10] Prime Minister David Cameron provided the observation that has become obligatory to such announcements—including those made by royals[11]—that mental health problems tend to be overlooked, and that too many suffer in silence.[12] Yet whilst it remains true that sometimes mental health problems are stigmatised and underdiagnosed, the argument that multitudes are therefore suffering in silence is increasingly untenable when it is a matter of record that a growing percentage of the population are being medicated and excused work.[13]

Not to be outdone by Cameron's initiatives, five months later his successor, Theresa May, announced on her first day in office that shortfalls in mental health services were one of the country's 'burning injustices'.[14] The following year, this was followed up with the promise of an extra 10,000 NHS mental health staff, one of those suspiciously round numbers so beloved of politicians seeking to make an impact.[15] Soon after, borrowing from the example of Royal Mail, it was promised that 'Mental Health First Aid' training would be made available to every secondary school in the country.[16] Not long after that, on A-Level results day, May announced another new course designed to raise awareness of mental illness amongst young people generally, notching up the anxiety surrounding the issue with reference to its potentially 'devastating effect'.[17]

Like Royal Mail and the makers of *The Secret Life of the Manic Depressive*, the government is sparing no effort in training people how to be ill. Some feel that it is doing too good a job of raising awareness. Notably, the first psychiatrist to be appointed as a president of the Royal Society of Medicine, Sir Simon Wessely, has been amongst the first to call publicly for an end to such campaigning: 'Every time we have a mental health awareness week my spirits sink. We don't need people to be more aware. We can't deal with the ones who already are aware.'[18]

As for diverting resources to mental health services, the objection is not the proposition that they are underfunded (like all parts of the health service) but the unquestioning way in which all additional spending is considered to be an appropriate prioritisation of scarce resources. Less trumpeted was the fact that, two months prior to Prime Minister May's promise of a further 10,000 mental health staff, the government had had to abandon its eighteen-week waiting time target for operations.[19] The presumptuous mindset that throwing more money at mental health services is the only possible answer restricts the issue to one of increasingly desperate supply-side solutions.[iii] It precludes more honest and contentious debate about the irresistible need, sooner or later, to contemplate how the demand is to be dialled down. Yet the mathematics are inevitable. The argument about the future funding of mental health services is a pregnant one but, as yet, very few wish to acknowledge the growing bump.

[iii] There are, of course, some demand-side solutions already being used in the healthcare system, such as the NHS' 'Make the Right Decision' poster campaign promoting self-care and pharmacist advice as an alternative to making a GP appointment. But these tend to be directed towards physical ailments rather than mental illness: the posters cite hangovers, grazed knees, sore throats and coughs as examples of conditions appropriate for self-care. In surgery waiting rooms, such posters invariably sit alongside others berating the waste and immorality of missed appointments. But patients may not appreciate the extent to which DNAs (Did Not Attends) are a welcome relief to their GPs, as a means of keeping up with their barely manageable workload—an example of an unofficial demand-side solution.

Stemming the tide of medicalisation is hard work, and for as long as the sea level continues to rise the economy risks being submerged. The desperate response of the UK government to this threat was predicted, with remarkable perspicacity, in 1971 by the Italian neuropsychiatrist Franco Basaglia. In *The Deviant Majority: The Ideology of Total Social Control*, he foresaw what would occur in industrialised societies as their diagnostic incontinence became progressively worse.[20]

In the early days of our industrialisation, as the medical guild was still becoming established and the process of turning people into patients was in its infancy, the sick were sufficiently rare that they were interesting curiosities. They were not in such numbers as to be a threat to the survival of wider society. They could even provide a dubious cottage industry: there was a booming trade in asylum tourism during this phase.[21] Basaglia anticipated that, as medicalisation gathers pace and a growing proportion of the population comes to be defined as sick, so the division between the sick and healthy becomes blurred. There is then the inevitable requirement, within an industrial society, to assert that maybe the sick have at least some degree of capacity for productivity. There are so many sick people that their participation in the industrial effort is a necessity if output is to be sustained. To facilitate this, where everybody is a patient to some degree and where patienthood might otherwise be seen as a reason not to work, the very act of wage labour must be depicted as being of therapeutic value.

This is exactly what has transpired. In 2005, thirty-four years after Basaglia's book was published, the government launched its 'Health, Work and Wellbeing' strategy in response to widespread concern about the extent of sickness in Britain in the late twentieth and early twenty-first centuries. Fittingly, given Basaglia's prediction of a convergence of medical and economic interests, this was a collaboration between the Department of Health and the Department for Work and Pensions. One of the first publications to arise from the collaboration, Dame Carol Black's 'Working for a Healthier Tomorrow', focused on the theme that many people who were currently sick—perhaps as many as half of the 2.6 million claimants of state sickness benefits—were capable of work, given the right support.[22] In 2011, the Black-Frost report similarly emphasised the therapeutic properties of employment.[23]

So far, and as envisaged by Basaglia, the attempts to mount a counteroffensive to medicalisation have been indirect. We have harried at the flanks, rather than mounting a full-frontal counterattack. Perhaps the day will come when there is wider recognition of medicalisation as the scourge that it is, and we will question the sense in categorising such a high proportion of the working population as sick. Until then, we shall continue to procrastinate, pondering such riddles as whether ill people remain able to work in an epoch when it takes very little to be considered ill.

12

DIAGNOSTIC INCONTINENCE

When there was deference to professionals generally, and they practiced with relative impunity, doctors in particular could be effective in their social function of signalling to wider society who should and who should not be accepted as being ill. This served to limit the number of ill people and to protect the interests of the most vulnerable. In this way the sickness genie was at least partially kept in the bottle, though the Schuster report details how, even over a century ago, doctors were far from reliable policemen.[1]

Through applying a brake to the proportion of people within society who can legitimately claim to be patients, doctors in theory ensure that the financial and emotional capital available for sick people is not squandered. When only a small proportion of the community is 'under the doctor', and there is confidence that doctors are judicious in accepting claims of illness, societal compassion fatigue is avoided. Such a system can be helpful even to those given short medical shrift. In a society that has maintained faith in its doctors as the arbiters of who is ill, their forceful persuasion of some individuals that they are well carries

141

power of reassurance and—for those becoming inclined to fret about their health—can have health-giving properties.

To be effective, these assurances must be confidently given. No-one wants to hear that they 'probably' aren't about to die. But confidence can be misplaced; the potential for missed and misdiagnosis always exists. Then the practitioner can expect publicity, litigation and the stocks. Doctors are undermined in performing this reassurance function in a society with unrealistic expectations of perfection, and when they fear that bad luck or the occasional human error will be mercilessly punished. This is a shame as, whilst no system is perfect, one in which doctors retain the trust and support of society in deciding who is ill has much to commend it.

The reality today is that claims to illness are widely believed to be inadequately tested.[2] Doctors are terrified of giving reassurance, in the knowledge that on the once-in-a-blue-moon occasion they are wrong they will be sued.[3] As a result, nearly everybody is purportedly ill in some way, and the currency of illness has been debased. The needs of the sickest are lost in the clamour and miasma of first-world ills. They are at risk of dismissive, cynical treatment from those who are themselves sick and tired of the enforced kindness that our culture requires them to demonstrate towards the 'ill'.

Similarly, a growing public perception that the courts may be too prepared to accept claims of illness can undermine trust and confidence in the rule of law. Despite having been convicted of twenty-one counts of parliamentary expenses fraud, in 2012 Labour MP Margaret Moran was spared jail after a judge ruled she was 'not fit mentally to defend herself', having heard psychiatric opinion that she was severely depressed. The judge concerned probably understated the strength of public sentiment when he remarked that 'There will inevitably be feelings among some that Mrs Moran has got away with it.' In giving evidence, one psychiatrist opined that he did not know 'whether it would be physically possible to remove her from her home without restraining her.' The situation was probably not helped, five days after the judge's acceptance that she was too depressed to attend court, by her demonstrable ability to attend a local pub.[4]

Ernest Saunders' apparent miraculous recovery from dementia made plenty of press in the 1990s. 'Deadly' Ernest had been sentenced to five years' imprisonment in 1990 as one of the 'Guinness Four', convicted of fraudulently manipulating the Guinness share price. In 1991 his sentence was halved when the Court of Appeal was persuaded that he was dementing, having heard evidence from a consultant psychiatrist who said that Saunders was unable to recall three numbers backwards or use a door. Four months after his release, he was consulting at a rate of £16,000 per month. On being seen retrieving cash from an ATM, one journalist who happened to be passing has recalled how she quipped, 'Having any problems remembering your pin number, Ernest?'[5]

Sometimes huge sums of money can be at stake according to whether bad character or illness is accepted as the explanation for poor behaviour. In one widely reported case, there was an unusually pugilistic end to a strategy meeting when the tired and emotional executive chairman of The Automobile Association—with alcohol and tranquilisers on board—submitted a fellow executive to a 'sustained attack' in the bar of a country hotel. Following dismissal for gross misconduct, he lost share options thought to be to the tune of £68 million. It was reported that his lawyers would litigate an unfair dismissal claim on the grounds that he had only beaten up his colleague due to the high pressure and stress of his role.[6]

The sexual peccadillos—or worse—of Hollywood actors and impresarios periodically surface in the media. It will then be a matter of nanoseconds before the paparazzi are treated to the spectacle of them lugubriously checking in to a rehabilitation clinic, grim-faced and shielded by sunglasses. But it is only a contrition of sorts. The intended public relations perception is of another fragile and flawed human preparing to battle their demons in the way that a cancer patient may steel themselves for the chemotherapy that must follow. The subtext being, 'it was not my fault, it was my unruly genitals or the faulty part of my brain that controls them—can you begin to imagine the living hell that is my sex addiction?' Even the American Psychiatric Association has yet to allow this expedient condition back into its hallowed and lengthening list of potential excuses for human misdemeanours (it was included in DSM-III in 1980, and removed from DSM-IV in 1994). It is probably just a matter of time.

This is the state of medicine today: generally, doctors are kept busy addressing the ills of people without any disease that exists irrefutably and in a measurable way,[i] with poorly effective treatments, in a hostile climate where they fear complaint and litigation, and occasionally embroiled in the affairs of characters pursuing their own social, contractual and legal agendas. As Aldous Huxley observed, men make use of their illnesses as much as their illnesses make use of them. Unsurprisingly, the plain speaking of Sir Lancelot Spratt-type characters is now largely the stuff of history.[ii] They could not afford the indemnity premium

---

[i] Malleson writes: 'there is no reason why a newly turned out doctor should be any better at curing colds ... than anybody else. He certainly has not learnt anything about the management of minor physical disorders, nor has he learned how to deal with embattled families and with human unhappiness. He soon learns from his patients.' (*The Medical Runaround*, p. 17.)

[ii] Sir Lancelot, the irascible yet confidence-inspiring general surgeon played by James Robertson Justice in a series of comedy films during the 1950s and '60s, spouted reassuring lines such as 'Don't be alarmed

their insurer would levy for a practitioner who routinely spoke their mind over appeasing the patient.

The medical consultation is now less a consultation, where the professional offers their unvarnished opinion in good faith and with the best interests of the individual in mind, and more like booking a holiday with a travel agent. The individual's assertion that they are ill is challenged no more than their expression of desire to take a holiday. Prospective tourists flick through the brochures and instruct the travel agent on where they would like to go and how they would like to get there. Today's patient is inclined to helpfully advise their doctor as to which specialist they should be referred to and what investigations should be ordered in the meantime. They may need a special visa arranged in preparation for their trip, the Med3 sick-note, and conveniently for them the doctor has a handy pile of these available.

Medicalisation is a tango: it takes two. Unfortunately, willing dance partners meet up all too often. People who do not tend to consult doctors and who are sceptical when they do cannot be medicalised easily, but they are increasingly in the minority. And although would-be patients cannot medicalise unless the doctor will anoint them with a diagnosis—rather than trying to reassure them that they are merely experiencing life's slings and arrows—generally that is exactly what will happen. Doctors medicalise out of naivety or self-interest. For some the urge to help is so strong as to be irrepressible, and it is a case of whacking away at screws with a hammer rather than admitting that they lack a screwdriver. In the main, it is self-preservation. Large numbers of patients with Shit Life Syndrome of varying severity beat a path to their door seeking a medical solution to their unsatisfac-

---

madam, I've removed hundreds of stones in my time. Enough to cobble a courtyard.'

tory circumstances.[7] It is more expedient for the doctor to connive than to engage in futile argument.

Sometimes there is an egotistical or pecuniary reason for medicalising. Careers can be made by subspecialisation in a controversial new illness, classically a 'medically unexplained syndrome' that reputable doctors remain reticent to acknowledge. Such controversy allows these panjandrums to depict themselves as enlightened and fearless to the criticism from their staid and heartless colleagues. This endears them all the more to their willing patients. The latter feel similarly estranged from the practitioners of mainstream medicine, who have failed to explain their symptoms to their satisfaction in a manner that appeals to their pseudoscientific prejudices.

Union representatives and lawyers regularly go 'doctor shopping', seeking a practitioner who will provide medical opinion favourable to the interests of their members and clients. Those inclined to medicalise and dramatise will find themselves on speed-dial and can develop a reliable revenue stream. When acting for the claimant, there is more money to be made by developing a reputation as an expert who consistently diagnoses a compensable medical harm than as one who describes hurt feelings, venting spleens and disjointed noses in plain English. Acting for the defendant, the best money is to be made if one is known to absolve people whose behaviour has been unequivocally bad, or sparing them the full weight of the law, on grounds of illness.

Since Britain's involvement in a series of bloody Middle Eastern conflicts since the 1990s—those in Iraq and Afghanistan in particular—there has been justifiable public concern over the mental health of veterans and of the potential for post-traumatic stress disorder in particular. There are those who fear that this has been exploited by some for commercial gain. Conservative MP Johnny Mercer, who himself completed three tours of Afghanistan and has spoken about his own, unrelated mental illness, condemned charities who 'have gone way too far in painting the picture of [PTSD among] veterans in the UK for their own ends, to raise money. They do it because they are a business, because they want the money.'[8] This from a man with a consistent and heartfelt commitment to the cause of veterans and the cause of mental health provision more generally, whose maiden speech to Parliament three years previously had focussed on the inadequate mental health treatment available to ex-combatants in particular.[9]

Sometimes the relationships between vulture-like doctors and lawyers feeding on medicolegal carrion can be especially close. In one instance, a court found that a young couple had fraudulently demanded thousands of pounds in compensation from the holiday operator TUI, for allegedly having their holiday ruined by food poisoning. TUI discovered that the doctor who had presented medical evidence on behalf of the couple was married to a partner in the law firm representing them. They took a dim view of what had the appearance of a cottage industry, reporting the doctor concerned to the General Medical Council and the legal firm to the Solicitors Regulation Authority.[10]

In the main, when patients medicalise inappropriately it is for the more prosaic reason that they are not managing their lives sufficiently well with the non-medical coping strategies at their disposal, and life as a patient seems preferable. In *The Last Well Person*, the American physician Nortin Hadler eloquently explains how, by and large, becoming a patient is more to do with healthcare-seeking behaviours than with having symptoms substantially worse than those of anybody else. Symptoms amongst 'well' people are so common as to be normal. If you consider yourself well, this fact may come as a surprise, because you may not consider yourself as someone especially prone to symptoms. That is because feeling well is largely synonymous with feeling invincible to a hostile and uncertain world. It means that, at the time we are experiencing unpleasant sensations—an ache, a spasm, trapped wind, a sudden pang of anxiety—we tend not to pay too much heed, as our confidence in our ability to endure and to come out the other side remains unshaken. Subsequently, we would not even recall the event unless some nosy parker with a clipboard stopped us in the street to ask us about it.

That is exactly what Nordic researchers did. Four thousand people were asked to recollect whether they had experienced any of ten common symptoms listed on the survey questionnaire over the preceding thirty-day period. More than 50% had experienced tiredness, 42% headache, 37% worry, 35% low back pain and 33% pain in their arms or shoulders. Over 75% of them reported having had at least one of those symptoms, and 52% had had two or more.[11]

The ill and the well are distinguished more by their psychosocial circumstances—the extent to which they feel in control and able to manage the hardships of their lives, and the degree of social and occupational support they feel they are receiving whilst doing so—than they are separated by their biology. With this insight, it is possible to see how symptoms are often merely the proverbial straw that breaks the camel's back. Illnesses are often symbolic, the hot water bottle and bed rest of the invalid a shorthand means of communicating to others that their wherewithal to cope is temporarily overwhelmed. The snag of medicalisation is that all attention is then focussed on the final straw, which is to miss the point that it is the heavy load of life that has brought the person to their knees. But medicalisation will remain with us for as long as people need to drape their suffering in the cloak of illness in order to elicit a sympathetic reaction from the outside world.

Doctors often recognise this, and it is perfectly possible to lack confidence that there will be a medical solution to a problem whilst also feeling compassion for the individual. The 'lethal paradox', as Malleson has coined it,[iii] is that doctors with the humility not to interfere in situations where they don't believe they can help are perceived as uncaring, whilst those prepared to rush in and dispense all manner of potentially dangerous treatments[iv] are merely perceived as unlucky when things don't work out.

In modern Western culture, as the medical consultation comes more closely to resemble booking a holiday than being bawled out by Sir Lancelot Spratt, it is the individual who decides if they are ill and, as Dr Handfield-Jones observed, whether they should go sick.[12] The doctor—often against their better judgement—merely suggests treatments they may wish to try, and provides the certificate. Once in this role, the individual is no longer a person in the normal sense, expected to demonstrate stoicism and personal responsibility for their own welfare, but instead a patient.

Fundamentally patienthood is a passive role;[v] the expectation of self-sufficiency is pleasantly alleviated. The subspecialisation of labour within industrialised society means that when somebody is ill we place the burden of responsibility for their recovery on the professionals. In this paradigm, the patient is the amateur. They are no more responsible for their own recovery than the householder is expected to know how to repair their broken-down boiler whilst waiting for the central heating engineer to arrive.

[iii] *The Medical Runaround*, p. 30.

[iv] All treatments are potentially dangerous, as to be effective they must be potent. If they did not have the potential to harm, they could not have the potential to cure. This places a sober responsibility on doctors to prescribe with caution, embodied in Hippocrates' primary instruction that, above all else, doctors should do no harm.

[v] The term 'patient' entered use in the 14th century from the Old French *pacient*, sharing the same root as 'passive': the Latin verb *patior* (past participle *passus*), meaning to bear, suffer or endure.

There was once the expectation that patients at least comply with 'doctor's orders' in order to get better. Today, even this obligation is liable to be excused, now that the traditional patient–doctor relationship is seen as overbearingly patriarchal and patronising. Protests of not wanting to be treated with anything 'unnatural' are fairly common. Nonscientific beliefs are prevalent in a medicalised society, and this attitude is often quite protective for the patient, although not for the reason they think. It isn't that prescription drugs and treatments are inherently bad, just that they are not ill enough in the first place to warrant taking any risks with them. The ambivalent patient, who has not thrown themselves wholeheartedly into the business of being ill, does tend to limit the doctor to the status of observer rather than practitioner, however. One then has to question what the point of the exercise is, other than to enjoy the status of patienthood.

Involving doctors in situations that are fundamentally not medical has predictably unsatisfactory, costly and harmful consequences. We can't afford for seriously ill people to be left loitering in surgery waiting rooms whilst the GPs busy themselves dispensing folk wisdom, amateur life coaching and cod psychology to those aggrieved by twenty-first-century life. It is the inalienable right of hairdressers, taxi drivers and publicans to perform these functions; doctors are interlopers who have intruded onto their turf, and with about as much qualification.

Being medicalised allows the person who previously had a life problem that was theirs to cope with to become a patient. They are thereby able legitimately to assume the sick role whilst waiting for their doctor to contrive a solution. This transfer of responsibility is comfortable enough for people who do not want to make the effort in, or take accountability for, the conduct of their own lives. Many may not even be aware that their locus of control is slipping externally to an unfeasible extent—such is the power of the subliminal conditioning associated with a medicalised society.[vi] Better still, if the medicalisation has been wholly inappropriate, and there are no effective treatments for the doctor to find, the wait—and the period of sick leave—will predictably be a long one. The skyrocketing rates of sickness absence due to work-related stress in recent years are the epitome of this phenomenon.[13] Stress is catching, and that is not surprising. With this condition employees can indulge themselves in vexed self-righteousness, not only at the indifference of their employer but at the uselessness of their doctor too.

Sometimes people medicalise in a lucid and deliberate way, for the reason John Stuart Mill described all those years ago: because they would be mugs not to. As we know (see Chapter 7), politicians spent the last few decades of the twentieth century encouraging uptake of sickness benefits for reasons of political expedience. People whose jobs in engineering, mining and heavy industry had evaporated were happy to oblige rather than residing on the dole. Perversely, even for those who do have jobs it often makes sense to medicalise rather than to manage. Within organisations that are dysfunctional, and unable to consistently manage incapability—especially when this is alleged to have a medical basis—employees feel they need to be ill simply to be treated fairly.

These employers are characterised by a disastrous combination of timorous management—senior managers who undermine junior managers' attempts to manage incapability, by failing to

---

[vi] The psychologist Julian Rotter coined the locus of control theory in the mid-50s. Those with an implausibly internal locus of control—perceiving their own decisions and actions as disproportionately important in their lives—struggle to adjust to unfortunate events, as a result of a misplaced sense of failure and guilt. Those with an excessively external locus are more inclined to sleepwalk through life, not asserting control to their fullest potential, because of a failure to appreciate their own agency.

support them when employees lodge tactical grievances—and a paranoid fear of occasionally having to account for their actions in tribunal. These obstructive policies have the effect of creating perverse incentives for disability among those who are not, in truth, medically disadvantaged against their peers. There is growing resentment on the part of those employees who perform hard, dirty or dangerous work without complaint and who feel increasingly exploited. None of this augurs well.

The essence of modern human resources theory is that maximising employee engagement is the Holy Grail of improved productivity. Unsurprisingly, people's sense of whether they are treated fairly is determinant of how committed they feel towards their employer.[14] This means that they think it is important that their efforts and contribution be recognised, and that crewmates who are not pulling hard enough on their oars—for whatever reason, whether lazy, exhausted or ill—be pulled up by the bosun. When employees perceive that this is not the case, they may feel that natural justice requires them to compromise their work ethic. According to the wisdom of John Stuart Mill, it would make more sense for them also to slump on their oars, rather than to persevere. Formerly motivated employees calculate—quite rationally—that it is not in their personal interest to endure aches, pains and discomforts without complaint while others are not doing the same, and observe that, conversely, exaggerating the extent of any symptoms they may have will tend to be rewarded.

In other words, employees in workplaces lacking fairness are understandably motivated to medicalise, and as a consequence a significant proportion of that workforce is either absent from work on oxymoronic 'stress leave' or, if in work, only fulfilling a proportion of the employment contract. Since people's illnesses these days are by and large what they say they are, the doctor's role being reduced essentially to note-taking, medicine provides little or no protection to organisations that are falling sick in this way. Employees who have feigned or embellished an illness to achieve a reward that will only be theirs for as long as they are sick have no intention of getting better.

The Metropolitan Police was singled out by Jerry Morris in his 1965 paper about the paradox of rising sickness rates in an era of improving healthcare. How has this organisation fared in the years since? Figures from 2016 reveal that, at any one time, 4.1% of officers are on sick leave, 3.4% are temporarily working less than full duties whilst easing back into work after illness, and 4.1% have a long-term exemption from normal operational duties in relation to an enduring disablement.[15] Thus, on any given day in our capital city, more than one officer in nine is either not on shift or at least unable to be deployed in the normal manner as a result of ill health, something that the press has reported with alarm.[16] The picture is similar across provincial forces and reported with similar concern in the local press from places such as Oxford and Nottingham.[17]

There are other bellwether signs that all is not well within the Met. In just three years, between 2010/11 and 2013/14, the number of days lost to stress-related sickness in particular rose by 53%, from 15,760 to 24,065—and the number of resignations, for those wanting to cut ties more comprehensively, rose by 62%, from 312 to 506.[18] Probably for complex reasons—perhaps because traditionally women have tended to shoulder a disproportionate share of family and caring responsibilities—the issues are especially acute amongst female officers across England and Wales. In 2016, 5.2% and 6% were on recuperative and restricted duties respectively, compared with 2.3% and 3.2% for their male counterparts.[19]

Royal Mail—then the Post Office—was the other employer specifically mentioned by Morris. Its sickness rates are similar to those of the Met, 4.63% for the year 2016/17.[20] Like most employers, Royal Mail does not conventionally report data about the proportion of staff who are in work but on modified duties, but its annual corporate responsibility report from this year states that approximately 7 per cent of staff identified themselves as 'disabled'. It seems likely that the proportion not working in their full role for reasons of illness is also roughly similar to that seen in the Met. It would be unfair to single out the Met and the Royal Mail, mentioned here for no other reason than their inclusion in Morris' 1965 paper, without saying that these are problems common to UK organisations in general and especially, in my experience, within the public sector and in large corporates.

After more than a decade as a medical advisor to police forces, I can attest that police work is hard work. Officers are subjected daily to abuse, hostility, intimidation and violence. They work in an environment of budgetary constraints and resource shortages, led by managers whose capacity to lead and maintain morale in challenging conditions is perpetually frustrated by the requirement for them to remain ever mindful of the extensive civilian employment law that now applies to police officers. I came to have enormous respect for the sense of vocation possessed by the great majority of police officers, and growing disdain for those politicians and policy-makers away from the frontline whose actions have made life so much more difficult for them.[vii]

[vii] The Disability Discrimination Act 1995 (the forerunner to the disability provisions of the Equality Act 2010) did not apply to police officers until 1 October 2004. The impact of such legislation on the civilian economy is discussed in later chapters. The time-consuming complexity of this law, and the effect it would have on operational effectiveness, means that the Armed Forces have always been exempt from it, although periodically it's suggested that this exemption be removed. In my experience, the requirement for police managers forever to contemplate how far

DIAGNOSTIC INCONTINENCE

Away from the station politics created by these civilian rules, officers are ground down by an increasingly toxic culture across some sections of society. This is characterised by institution-alised grievance, antagonism towards the police, impossible expectations of perfection and tactical allegations of police brutality from repeat offenders who are regularly detained and know the drill.[21] Officers attend work each day in the knowledge that, should anybody come to harm as a result of their (non-)exercise of their powers, they will be subject to a gruelling, public, retrospective investigation of their actions in minute detail in the tabloid court of public opinion.

Behind the force-level statistics, there will be human stories. But whatever is happening at the level of the individual—whether the disablement is unavoidable or a calculated survival tactic—there can be little doubt that organisations with these levels of absence and disability have themselves become sick.

---

they should modify roles in order to accommodate legally disabled officers (with bad backs or anxiety, for example) is diametrically opposed to the decisions they must regularly make in order to maintain morale and operational effectiveness within what is at times a paramilitary service, in an age of constant terrorist threat. During my time with police, it was apparent that much management practice is very poor, but I came to be persuaded that this is often because the objectives managers are set are hopelessly conflicted.

THE WORKPLACE AND THE LAW

13

CONSENTING ADULTS

As the single greatest cause of sickness absence, accounting for almost half of lost days, stress warrants especial scrutiny.[1] The solutions to the stress epidemic are not difficult to fathom. They are, however, unpalatable and awkward to implement, at a time when many employers have unwisely put themselves in a double bind by buying quite so enthusiastically into the 'wellbeing' agenda of recent years.

In promoting the lie that the welfare of staff is their 'primary' concern, businesses have further confused those employees who already have an unrealistic expectation of the employer's role as nursemaid in their lives. They have written cheques they cannot cash. The prevailing sense of entitlement has been potentiated, and now manifests more frequently in the form of employment disputes and absenteeism. This is in the same way that the correct mix of meteorological conditions can precipitate a downpour out of humid air.

When a police force asked me to comment on a mental health strategy it had developed for its police officers, including declarations of intent such as 'your health is our first concern', I complained bitterly—and to little effect—that this was liable to backfire. Surely, I reasoned, policing the streets was the first concern of a police force—with the noble goal that, whilst doing so, the force might also aspire at least to minimising the health risks to its officers, as far as it could? Otherwise the best course of action would be to confine all officers to their station and let the citizenry duke it out amongst themselves.

This was a period when, as a result of terrorist attacks, all forces were anxious about the potential for marauding attacks, following the 2008 terrorist co-ordination of twelve shootings and bombings in Mumbai over a four-day period. In 2017, British officers did indeed need to respond to similar 'roving' atrocities, at Westminster Bridge (March) and London Bridge (June). Such attacks represent a very different tactical challenge from IRA bombings, for instance. Now, unarmed officers in the wrong place at the wrong time—or in the right place at the right time, depending on perspective—are expected to confront moving and multiple threats as best they can.[i] All sensible officers appreciated this, only the jejune ones did not. Thus the net effect of this 'health first' strategy and its fatuous platitudes was to disenfranchise the majority, by appearing disingenuous, and to exacerbate the existing tendency of a minority of malcontents to feel hard done by each and every time they were deployed into harm's way.

---

[i] This public expectation of unquestioning and ultimate sacrifice from the police was demonstrated by the fierce criticism of Sir Craig Mackey during the inquest into the Westminster Bridge attack. The deputy commissioner had remained in his car while an unarmed officer was stabbed to death, because he had no protective equipment and no radio. Although Mackey could in no way have altered events, except perhaps by adding his own life to the fatalities, the *Daily Express* ran a headline declaring the victim a 'Police hero who put his boss to shame'.

Contrary to much current thought, roles exist within an organisation solely because they are necessary in order for its objectives to be realised. In most organisations, the stakes are lower than the life-and-death responsibilities of a police force and instead these objectives are about the commercial survival of a business. But the principle is the same: the needs of the individual are subservient to those of the organisation. In a capitalist free-market economy, the principle role of business—its raison d'être, no less—is to be profitable for its shareholders, and thereby to remain capitalised and in business. For the public sector, it is to honour its fiduciary duty to the taxpayer to deliver public services in the most cost-efficient manner.[ii]

It is not the task of the public sector, nor of business, to engage in some deluded experiment in central planning, seeking purposefully to create employment surplus to requirements; nor to design jobs with the express intention of making people happy. Full employment is the remit of dictators, laughter the remit of comedians; neither are the responsibility of business-owners or those paid to orchestrate the efficient delivery of public services. In the 1930s, the Canadian politician William Aberhart learnt from a foreman that there was a deliberate policy of building airports with picks and shovels rather than heavy plant, so as to maximise the number of construction jobs created. He suggested that if the object of the exercise was to lengthen out the task, the foreman should go further and provide the workers with spoons and forks.[2]

[ii] In his foreword to a 2013 publication by HM Treasury, 'Managing Public Money', Danny Alexander (then chief secretary to the Treasury) explains how—if it is to retain credibility with taxpayers—government must be able to demonstrate that it spends taxes wisely, and that this is a thread that can be traced back through the Bill of Rights to *Magna Carta*.

In the same vein, the modern concern is that automation and robotics may do away with a great many of the jobs that currently exist. The extraordinary efficiencies of machine-learnt artificial intelligence and robotics will be irresistible to business. Thought is already being given to taxing robot-owners in order to generate compensation for those left workless as a result, in the form of a general basic income.[iii] Forced human employment in these circumstances will appear as Luddite to modern eyes as expecting construction workers to work with shovels did to Aberhart. In a free society where no-one is compelled to offer employment for the sake of it, jobs exist for a purpose and not as an end in themselves. Where evolving economic needs in the imminent robot economy generate demand for new jobs requiring qualities of humanity and creativity, rather than monotonous toil—in other words, better jobs—then that is all to the good. But these are fortuitous byproducts of capitalism, not its central objective. The labour market is not a component part of a Soviet state, nor is it a national daycare clinic for occupational therapy, however much it may sometimes feel like that.

Adam Smith encapsulated this notion that capitalism can be a means of providing efficiently for society, but only when it is first satisfying its own ends: 'It is not from the benevolence of the butcher, the brewer, or the baker that we expect our dinner, but from their regard to their own interest.' Maybe this is not the best possible way of ordering our society, but the United Kingdom is a democracy where political parties are free to pro-

---

[iii] This was first a suggestion of Mady Delvaux, a socialist Luxembourgish MEP, in a May 2016 European Parliament report. It has subsequently been proposed by other European socialist leaders including the French politician Benoît Hamon and Britain's Jeremy Corbyn, as well as by Microsoft founder Bill Gates—whose products will have displaced many clerics and administrators from work in an earlier wave of automation.

pose alternatives and, as yet, voters have not chosen to disrupt the status quo. It is a reasonable conclusion, therefore, that, for the majority at least, this is the preferred way of doing things— however much they may grumble when things do not go their way. This is probably because the accoutrements of an industrialised world—shiny cars and shinier gadgets—appeal more to most than rustic simplicity. We prefer to keep up with the Joneses (these days, the Kardashians) rather than the Goods.[iv] Currently, and until the electorate chooses otherwise, the rat race is the way that we do things. It is the basis on which individuals enter into contracts of employment with their employer. These are not altruistic arrangements, but mutually beneficial ones.

Some people's experience of employment is terrifying and distressing, as a result of treatment meted out to them at work. Intimidating, harassing and bullying behaviour occurs in the workplace as everywhere else where human beings congregate. Such scenarios are better thought of as being distressing rather than stressful. They are the concern of everyone in the organisation who is aware of what is happening, especially management and—in larger companies—the human resources team. There is no medical solution to such abuses any more than there is to mugging. The issues are moral and legal, and they require policing and the dispensation of justice. Employers must exercise their duty of care to their employees through creating a culture of mutual respect and fairness, and by following their policies and procedures relating to equality and diversity, dignity at work, whistleblowing, grievances, misconduct and the like. Arbitrating such disputes can be a nightmarish distraction from the actual

---

[iv] The 1970s sitcom *The Good Life* tapped into the disillusionment many people feel with life in a consumer society. The central characters, Tom and Barbara Good, tried to escape commercialism by converting their suburban home into a self-sufficient smallholding.

job of work, but it is also a cost of doing business in a civilised society. Wherever there are groups of people there will be interpersonal disputes, some real, some perceived, all of which need to be managed.

When the employer's internal processes are insufficient to satisfy the individual, then these problems become a matter for the employment tribunals and courts. These are not cases that relate to some dispute about the employment contract, but instead to allegations of inherently unreasonable behaviour. In our society—thankfully—we would not accept as lawful a contract which expressly or implicitly set an expectation that an employee might be maltreated by management, and so should suck it up. People turning up for work are entitled to hope that they will not be verbally or physically attacked on entering the foyer, or indeed by their executive chairman at the bar after a strategy meeting.

In the main, when people talk about stress, and specifically work-related stress, they mean something other than the distress of people who feel bullied and harassed. They are talking about situations where the different parties to the employment contract have different expectations of it, and where friction is generated as a result. Stress has been conceptualised in various ways. Commonly it is defined as the subjective, unpleasant experience of an individual when they feel that demands being placed on them are outstripping their capacity to cope.

Again, as with behavioural standards, the employer has a duty in terms of how the contract is enacted. The employee can have the reasonable expectation that their employer—personified in the form of the manager—will engage in conversation with them if there are any aspects of their job which are proving difficult, or where they may benefit from some additional training, tools or collegiate support. Thereafter, though, things become a little trickier. Even if it is accepted that, to use the legalese, the 'provisions, criteria and practices' of the role are placing the employee under strain—and even making them feel unwell—it does not necessarily follow that the employer has done anything wrong, nor that there is necessarily an onus on them to intervene.

Logically, there can be one of two explanations why the employee may feel this way. It may be that the expectations for the role—in terms of the output that is expected from them, with the resources and supports that the employer feels they can provide—are fair, but that the employee is incapable of meeting them. Or, it may be that the expectations for the role are unreasonable. The problem, of course, is in deciding which is which.

In Shakespeare's *The Merchant of Venice*, the title character, Antonio, contracts with the miserly moneylender Shylock. The nature of the arrangement is that, if a loan made by Shylock is not repaid, he will be entitled to a pound of Antonio's flesh. There are many themes to the play, and the protagonists are multifaceted. Shylock is a vengeful and vindictive character, seeking to pursue his contract to the letter, even if the cutting of his pound of flesh should mean the death of Antonio. He is deaf to attempts to renegotiate the original arrangement in a way that would actually be to his advantage. Antonio's peril tends to attract our sympathy, but, nevertheless, the reality is that he has welched on a deal—one he cavalierly entered into of his own volition. Neither are especially attractive characters. The employment tribunals are rammed with modern-day Shylocks and Antonios.

Except in extreme cases, it is impossible to say definitively whether or not a role is reasonable. The answer will always be that 'it depends'. It may be that the work is difficult, arduous, dirty, demands antisocial hours or is even dangerous. But it may also be that the terms and conditions offered by the employer in question are the going rate for that kind of job. In which case, who is anyone to dictate to the employer that they should pay more or expect less, and in so doing put them out of business altogether, or at least reduce the number of workers they can afford to employ? Many years ago, as a new occupational physician, one of the first cases I was asked to assess was a man who worked as a standby jet engineer. In the event that an airliner were stranded, he could be summoned at short notice to fly to inhospitable parts of the world, where he would be expected to work tirelessly until the defective engine was serviceable again. Listening to his miseries at the hands of his wicked employer was enough to almost move me to tears. Until, that is, I later learnt that the remuneration for his martyrdom was a quarter of a million pounds per annum.

Defining what is or is not a reasonable role requires a value to be put on the proverbial pound of flesh that the employer seeks to extract: the employee's time, and the hardships they will encounter whilst working. Different people will attach different financial values to the same work. In countries with pitifully low living standards, people will work for a pittance. The sewage workers of Delhi wallow in the city's sewers to clear blocked drains for £3.50 per day, presumably because the alternative of not working is even worse.[3] Conversely, when there is a benefits safety-net then unpleasant work—such as the back-breaking labour of picking fruit and crops—is unlikely to appeal.[4] Free movement of labour means that people more desperate for work may arrive from thousands of miles away, whilst the indigenous population put their feet up to Judge Rinder.

Providing it is lawful and compliant with all relevant statute relating to terms and conditions, any given job cannot be pronounced unequivocally unreasonable according solely to its productivity expectations.[v] It depends what pay is being offered to undertake it and, for those declining the work, what alternatives are on offer. There are some jobs that practically no-one would

---

[v] See, for example, the Working Time Regulations 1998 and the Management of Health and Safety at Work Regulations 1999.

perform for the minimum wage, and some jobs that nearly anyone would tolerate for £1 million per annum. The instrument for price discovery in terms of the value of a job is the free movement of labour within the jobs market. If the employer cannot recruit and retain, then the job is too arduous and unpleasant for the pay offered; if there is a queue snaking out of the recruitment office, then the pay offered is too much. Crudely and broadly, if an employer cannot fill a post, it is difficult to dispute that the market has spoken and the terms are unreasonable. If there is no such difficulty, then the market has delivered a different message. This is especially true during periods of low unemployment, as at the time of writing (October 2018), when unemployment is at its lowest for over forty years, and there is no body of unemployed workers large enough to depress wages.[5]

Of course, things are not quite so simple. It may be a false economy for the employer to offer pay and rations that are sufficient to recruit but not to retain, especially in roles where there is an investment in training a technical skillset. Or, the employer may judge that demonstrating goodwill and paying slightly more than the going rate will be reciprocated in terms of better productivity. But, in either case, the value attached to the role is still determined by the business case and not emotively. When all is said and done, the value of the job on the open market is still quantified in pounds and pence.

Where nuance does exist within assessments of how reasonable a job might be, it can be found in how the role is undertaken, rather than in the expectations for output and the pay that is offered. Some managers have a streak of Shylock's unyielding desire to enforce the letter of the contract in the face of all reason and common sense, and even to their own detriment. They enjoy the power afforded by their position to deny perfectly reasonable—or even mutually advantageous—requests that the employee has made. These may be about different ways of achieving the same objective, perhaps more efficient ones, or requests for training and support which, in the great scheme of things, are really no skin off the manager's nose. The driver for this behaviour may be sheer pettiness, born of a desire to assert the inviolable power balance of the relationship (in which the manager instructs, and the employee does). Such managers can assure themselves that it is they who occupy the moral high ground. After all, and like Shylock, they merely want their pound of flesh—and no more, no less. Or it may be sadism, the pleasure of exercising this power to disappoint the employee, even if the latter's resultant absence or resignation makes things harder for the manager in the long run.[vi]

Sometimes the managers of sick organisations are simply ground down. Any ounce of human sympathy they once had has been wrung from them by the relentless demands for special favours from a medicalised workforce that sees these as their entitlement. They are reluctant to talk to employees, to find out what is difficult and what they could do to help, for fear of opening Pandora's box. If they encouraged employees to ask for help, they would then need to invest further time and effort in deciding whether what was being asked for was reasonable, which itself is an unappealing Catch-22. If they acquiesced, they fear they would be accused by their managers of being too soft, and thereby letting departmental performance targets slip. If they refused, they fear an employee's grievance or tribunal submission, and the criticism of their managers for being too intransigent and unreasonable. Being unapproachable is a survival tactic.

[vi] A variant of 'Now I've Got You, You Son of a Bitch!', one of the games described in the psychiatrist Eric Berne's seminal book *Games People Play* (1964), which uses the psychoanalytic theory of transactional analysis to describe stereotypical 'games' played out between people in different states of emotional maturity.

CONSENTING ADULTS

An employee's report that they are stressed by their job signifies, in and of itself, just one thing: they assess that the demands of the job are straining their coping mechanisms, and perhaps to an extent that they feel ill as a result. They are not always blaming their employer for this: it might be the gig to which they knowingly signed up, and there may be no hard feelings. It may be that the employee is quite satisfied with this state of affairs, and was anticipating such hardship as the cost of their sizeable pay-packet. Within the Square Mile, such stories are swapped as a badge of honour, without any insinuation of exploitation and certainly no desire for the lucrative arrangement to change. These workers bear their stress as an inevitable occupational hazard just as—at the other end of the income scale—the construction workers erecting skyscrapers all around them expect to have back pain. All these people are consenting adults and free, within reason, to choose how much they wish to trade the health of their bodies and minds in the grubby exchange for cash.

Normally, though, and outside of astronomically well-paid jobs, the complaint of stress is a loaded one. People generally report stress for a reason: there is the expectation of a response from the employer. For less confident managers, the 'S' word can evoke a Pavlovian fear response of wariness and confusion. Ideally, how should they react? Logically, the first response should be to establish what the problem is, and what the employee is seeking to have done about it. If the manager judges that the expectations for the role are unreasonable, or that more could reasonably be done to support the employee in meeting them, then the employee's 'illness' is not solely the employee's problem. They are merely the canary in the mine.

Alternatively, it may be that the expectations for—and circumstances of—the role are eminently reasonable. The manager has done all they reasonably can to help the employee to meet them, including consideration of any suggestions from the employee about alternative ways they could achieve the objectives for the role. In this case, conceptualising the stressed employee's symptoms as an illness is to miss the point. Instead, the issue is that the employee is poorly suited to the demands of the job. Then, what management action is appropriate depends on whether the employee feels stressed but is nevertheless an adequate performer, or whether they have good cause to feel anxious about their ability to do their job.

Some employees consistently and grossly underperform in their contractual work, but may never experience a moment's stress in their job. They are so lacking in insight as to the depth of their incapability, or so unappreciative of the organisation's expectations for their role, that the feeling of failure to cope is never engendered in them. Conversely, their more neurotic, perfectionist peers may invariably exceed all performance expectations in their work, in tasks that are comfortably within their competence, yet feel consistently stressed because of the exceptionally high performance expectations that they set themselves, or their nagging self-doubt as to their abilities.

The employment relationship is now so heavily legalised, as well as medicalised, that I have seen employers become paranoid about a perceived breach in their duty of care to these perfectionists in allowing them to continue working. This may partly be because stress is such a difficult concept to incorporate into policy and guidance, and careless use of language can generate much misunderstanding. Take, for example, the advice of an 'influential HR specialist' on the Chartered Management Institute's website: that employers have a duty to provide a 'stress-free place of work'.[6] How realistic an expectation can that ever be?

There is a danger that confused, absolutist messaging of this kind will over-sensitise the manager into thinking that, since the employee finds their work distressing, there is an onus on the employer to prevent them from continuing in the role. This is partial logic, but it does not cater for the ethical principle that, within reason, people are free to conduct their lives as they wish; nor for the fact that dismissing people tends to be fairly detrimental to their health and wellbeing too. It would be rum to dismiss an employee who was evidently stressed to the eyeballs by their work but who nevertheless wished to continue doing it, unless the impact on their health was so great that they were no longer able to function in the position. In that case, the problem has become one of capability rather than duty of care anyway.

Sensible employers should be loath to lose these diligent, high-performing individuals. The obvious approach, once the duty-of-care bogeyman has been exorcised, is to reassure and encourage the individual as far as possible—notwithstanding that worriers will always worry, at least a little. In these situations, employers should not be concerned that they will be held liable for allowing the neurotic employee to work, any more than they should feel vulnerable to criticism for employing people who have asthma, diabetes or epilepsy.

It is quite different when the employee's stress is well founded. The reality may be that the employee is indeed falling far short of what is needed, and that their stress is the manifestation of them having marked their own homework. This is a situation of incapability, pure and simple—just one into which the employee in question has acute and painful insight. A decisive capability process is going to be in everyone's interests. Yet, bizarrely—or perhaps not in such a medicalised and legalised environment—management may demur from progressing the capability process if there are fears that it is making the individual ill. But, unsurprisingly, people who cannot cope with the pressures of their own job are likely to cope poorly with the strain of a capability process too. I recall being left speechless on hearing a sobbing police officer, captured in a performance management initiative that had been launched across his force, complaining that the problem with his employer was that 'You're not allowed to be shit any more.' Well, quite.

The underlying issue in such cases is one of incapability, except doubly so. The individual is incapable, by their own admission, of the job which their employer has retained them to perform—or, at least, incapable of doing it without feeling intolerable strain. Not only that, assuming that their manager has been supportive and flexible where they can, this employee seemingly lacks the skills needed to negotiate this awkward turn of affairs with management without the issue becoming unhelpfully medicalised. All roads lead to Rome and, in situations like this, all attempts to analyse and discover the root cause of the problem lead to incapability. That may be incapability in the job, incapability to cope with the performance processes the employer deems necessary to help them perform in the job, or both.

Sometimes employers and lawyers become bogged down in surreal debates about how much of the employee's distress relates to their incapability for their role, and how much to difficulties—self-inflicted or otherwise—in their personal life, as though that could ever be measured, or indeed as though it matters. This is an absurd diversion. It is a mindset that assumes the employee has been wronged, and then sets about apportioning blame on that basis. It is like deciding the magnitude of a defendant's guilt according to how upset their alleged victim is, and whether the accuser is suggesting that there are others who should also cop some of the blame for the victim's feelings.

Misery loves company and often, when an employee portrays their manager as the villain in their life, there will be a supporting cast comprising an acrimonious ex, a new partner who doesn't understand them, and a credit card debt that was somehow someone else's fault: the assorted roadkill of a life's poor driving. In any sane world, attempts at quantifying the magnitude of the employer's tort would only begin once it was first established that there had even been a tort in the first place. The employer should stand or fall solely according to the evidence of how reasonable and flexible they have been in trying to help the employee perform the role. What matters is the business case of the employee's complaint against what action the employer took and why—recorded contemporaneously in the personnel file—not how the employee felt about the situation, or what soap-operatic twists and turns their personal life was taking. In the febrile politics of stress, there is little room for such logic.

It is better for everyone that incapability is managed, and it is vital that the process is not stalled by the employee's anguish. Peeling off the plaster cannot be considered kinder than doing what needs to be done without inordinate delay. Delaying the break-up with an ill-suited partner for reasons of pity rarely works out for the best. When stressed employees are justifiably stressed, because they are incapable, it is cruel to leave the sword of Damocles suspended over them for any longer than is considered polite or required by employment legislation. Generally, though, there is an aversion to 'shooting the Labrador', as the task is distastefully known amongst more battle-hardened human resources personnel.

Ironically, it is the incapable and resistant employees whom employers often make the most contorted efforts to retain in some capacity, probably out of fear of 'a scene' or of litigation. In contrast, employees who have the emotional maturity to accept with equanimity that they are a square peg in a round hole tend to exit fairly swiftly and quietly—during a flatlining performance process, by mutual agreement, or by resignation—and employers tend to let them go. Yet, notwithstanding any shortcomings in their technical aptitude for the job they originally applied for, this surely is the strength of character and adult behaviour that the employer should prefer to retain if possible, if there were another role available that was a better match for their skillset. The different treatment of those distressed by their incapability, as distinct from the merely incapable, is an instance of the squeaky wheel tending to get the grease.

In the final analysis, when an employee reports feeling stressed by their job and is expecting something to change, only the employer can decide whether the issue is one of organisational oversight or employee incapability. Until it has taken a position, it cannot possibly know what the appropriate response should be, as the options are diametrically opposite. If the problem is with the role, such as a pedantically inflexible management approach to its execution, then the employee requires a rapid apology, reassurance and promises of change; and all should be well. Alternatively, if the employer is satisfied that the role and its management are satisfactory, then the problem instead lies with the employee.

Effective and appropriate management of the stressed employee, then, is utterly dependent on the employer reaching a view as to whether the problem is with the individual or the organisation. Like a hopeless teenage crush, at some point there needs to be an 'It's not me, it's you' conversation—or vice versa. Yet, in my experience, management very rarely has the courage of its convictions to reach such a decision in a timely way. Instead procrastination is the order of the day whilst the duality of these two separate universes—one requiring a swift apology, one a swift capability process—is maintained. This is employment relations Schrödinger-style. Everyone's frustration and distress mounts whilst they are parked in purgatory.

14

STRESSFUL EXPERTS

If management does not know what to do with the stressed employee, where else might it look for direction? Commonly the employee will be directed to a confidential counselling service funded by the employer. These Employee Assistance Programmes (EAPs) have much to commend them as an accessible portal for anguished employees. Typically they are staffed by trained counsellors rather than people who profess to any higher level of expertise. Fortunately, speaking to people who have the outlook of an emotionally intelligent human being, rather than that of an expert, is very helpful. Often it is enough to steer the person away from looming patienthood and back into difficult, but necessary, conversation with their employer.

Sometimes though, the emotionality of the individual results in escalation—first to a psychologist, in turn perhaps a psychiatrist. This is especially so in circumstances where the employee has private medical insurance and the barrier to seeing a psychiatrist is low. This is in contrast to the risk-based rationing system in operation on the NHS, where only those in the most acute distress are likely to be seen. These can be horrendous situations as the employer's resolve to do what is needed softens with each escalation and, by implication, the employee comes to be perceived as more ill. In a parallel universe where they had already been freed from their contractual shackles, and were progressing in a new role to which they were better suited, the employee might already be well on the road to recovery instead.

But Malleson's 'lethal paradox' is at play. To divert the individual onto the healthier path, the clinician would need the humility and the confidence to recognise that this is not a problem that will benefit from medicalisation. They would need to say that they don't think the person will benefit from the kind of help they can offer, and that therefore they can't help—which is too difficult for many helpers to say. Instead, to alleviate their own anxieties about being blamed, which are generally around the risk of suicide, the clinician often does the opposite: ratcheting the tension up a notch to justify passing the case upwards. Melodramatic expressions of concern and hoovering up the individual into the mental health services will always be perceived as caring and appropriate, rather than cloying and unhelpful.

Yet people who are convinced that the root cause of the problems in their life exists in the shape of their manager, and not in their mind, make poor candidates for psychological and psychiatric approaches. And in a free society, short of restraining everyone who is going through a difficult phase in their life, the risk of suicide is never zero and always difficult to predict, even amongst people with no mental illness. The clinician's urge to medicalise may cause a great deal of harm by perpetuating the person's distress for weeks, months or, in some cases, years.

The American philosopher Nicholas Butler said that an expert is someone who knows more and more about less and less, until eventually they know everything about nothing. My experience is that the extent to which cases of work-related stress become medicalised, and the specialisation of the clinicians becoming involved, is inversely correlated with the probability of the practitioner providing sensible, practical advice as to what should be done about it. By the time that apex predator of the stress food chain, a private psychiatrist, is involved, there is often little hope of a successful rehabilitation. It is not that psychiatric interventions are inherently ineffective. It is that there is an elephant in the room—a breakdown in the employment relationship, probably irretrievable by that stage—because it is self-evident that relationship problems tend not to be amenable to psychiatric treatment.

Perhaps, in rare cases, a medical solution will eventually emerge, and it will become clear with hindsight that the employee's incapability and associated stress were in fact the product of a significant, underlying and undiagnosed psychiatric condition. Looking for such problems is the other reason sometimes given for the upward referral of such cases, but it tends to be a specious one. Overwhelmingly, such buck-passing indicates a lack of confidence in confronting the real problem, which is generally obvious. When someone protests that they cannot bear their manager, they are unlikely to be confabulating.

In 2008 Gordon Waddell, Kim Burton and Nicholas Kendall, who rank amongst the most respected researchers in the field of vocational rehabilitation,[i] undertook a comprehensive meta-analysis. They collated the findings of multiple studies that had investigated the effectiveness of return-to-work interventions. One of their conclusions was that, whilst there is good evidence that treatments for mental illness are clinically beneficial, 'There is no high quality evidence on the cost-effectiveness of interventions to improve work outcomes for common mental health problems'.[1] In other words, tinkering with people's brains and minds often changes how they feel, but it would be a mistake to

---

[i] Defined as 'whatever helps someone with a health problem to stay at, return to and remain in work.'

assume that it is therefore helpful in returning them to work. This is likely to be for the simple reason that these absences are often the result of a problem that is not medical but contractual. Unless the practitioner has a wand that can make either the incapability or the unreasonable manager disappear in a puff of smoke, the rest of their kit bag is going to be redundant.

For most of those patients whose incapability reaches the dizzy heights of psychiatric medicalisation, the destination, insofar as their employment is concerned, remains unchanged—but the journey there is that much more protracted and painful. For these people, Mental Health First Aiders and EAPs can be gateway drugs, encouraging a progression onto the harder drug of psychology and, in some cases, the really hard stuff of Class A private psychiatry. Escaping the clutches of the dealers may be their best hope.

The general practitioner will invariably be of little help to those employers who find it difficult to maintain warm relations with their employees. Whether the underlying problem is one of poor management, or an excessively entitled employee, the GP is not in a position to know and is unlikely to care,[2] and their response will be the same. They will dutifully side with their patient and reflect the latter's wishes to the employer.

From a gamesmanship point of view, acting as the patient's secretary is the only rational approach open to the GP. As we have seen, it is in the doctor's interests for patients to be kept onside, especially those of a disagreeable and complaining disposition. The latter may be regular visitors to the surgery for years to come, reattending after each minor or major upset in their life, and it is better for the doctor not to stray into their crosshairs as a co-accused—which is what will happen if they give any appearance of siding with the manager, or even of objectivity. If management are sufficiently offended and outraged by the doctor's attempts at conflict resolution, then they are unlikely to solicit further opinions from them, which is secretly what the doctor desires anyway. They drop the crockery in the manner of a surly twelve-year old who does not want to be asked a second time to help with the washing up. The GP is not about to play devil's advocate and deliver a treatise on the free market economy to a quarrelsome employee on behalf of the employer.[3]

Hence, in many cases, for those employers with access to one, the occupational physician will be summoned to adjudicate. The principled and logical position for them is to advise the employer that, medically, it is inadvisable for people to remain in circumstances that are distressing them for any length of time, but that as the underlying problem itself is contractual and not medical they are acting *ultra vires* if they attempt to prescribe how the dispute should be resolved. They can have no greater insight into the causes of the situation, purely from assessing the individual, than anyone else. What is needed is a management investigation into the employee's concerns, not a medical consultation, and then a management decision as to what should be done about them.

For all the occupational physician knows, the employee may be as lazy and incompetent as Homer Simpson. Or they may be industrious and saintly but unlucky enough to have landed themselves a neglectful or disinterested manager, or a Shylock: one of the low-grade psychopaths who infest the management chain in the same way as they are found in every other walk of life. Either way, beyond a listening ear and encouragement to take charge of their life, medicine has little to offer; any more than the doctor would presume to prescribe divorce or enforced reunion if the quarrel were matrimonial rather than contractual.

Sympathy, normalisation, reassurance and advice about the importance of communication with the employer are all humane and reasonable responses for the doctor to display to the stressed employee. Ill-conceived attempts at management consultancy, defining for the employer how the terms and conditions of employment should be modified so as to make the individual happy, are not. Yet prescriptive advice as to how the employee's role should be amended—in a manner that is more to their liking—is offered all too often by doctors prepared to blunder into these spats between consenting adults, who are parties to an employment contract, under the guise of 'medical advice'. These are operational, contractual instructions as to how one party would like the contract to operate. They only constitute medical recommendations in the semantic sense that they emanate from doctors. It is ridiculous to consider them as such, any more than the suggestion from a medically qualified neighbour to prune one's roses could be thought of as medical advice. GPs—who have to maintain long-term relationships with their patients, have other fish to fry, and for whom it can therefore be expedient to prostitute their medical credentials in this way—can be forgiven. Occupational physicians, temporarily parachuted in as the supposed experts, cannot. Yet frequently they too will fail to recognise when they have strayed from medical territory and into the minefield of employment relations.

Employers daft enough to rely on these doctors as their unofficial management consultants find this approach convenient enough in the short term. As a means of avoiding having to make management decisions for themselves, and as a totemic demonstration of 'care', this strategy can work for a time. But, in the longer term, a wider sickness takes hold. Other employees may be motivated to seek similarly expedient medical support, greater unfairness is then created, and the race to the bottom begun in earnest. When the fever reaches its peak, such a doubly user-friendly service—for both hopeful employees and their submissive managers—will keep the medical advisor providing it frenetically occupied with appeasing increasingly emboldened demands. The clinician may see this as no bad thing if they are being contracted on an item-of-service basis. Whether it is a good thing for anyone else is a different matter.

Whether it is the general practitioner, an occupational physician or indeed a psychologist or psychiatrist who has become involved, this doctor is neither the employee's mother nor the company's human resources director. This is a fight in which they have no dog. It may be that the employee's work is unavoidably difficult, dangerous, demoralising, dirty or dispiriting; it may also be that the pay and terms offered by the employer represent the fair market rate for doing it. If not, market forces and the free movement of labour are the ways in which the employer should be brought to see the error of their ways, and not the chiding of doctors.

Generally, when someone is sick and tired of their job, the answer is not elusive, but it requires everyone to make hard choices. The stressed employee must choose whether the desire to possess material wealth, if it means running with the other rats, trumps the wish for a peaceful life—if the price of that is having to live in a yurt. It is iPads, widescreen televisions, holidays to Mexico and German cars, or it is hair-plaiting and horticulture in the kibbutz. Either is a principled position, but to want both is hypocrisy. More charitably, if there are altruistic reasons why an employee feels compelled to remain in a situation that is proving toxic—as might be true for many Met officers, for example—then it is a choice between selflessness or self-interest. One has particular moral merit, and one is pragmatic. Again, there is not a third option of having both. Those who consciously choose the higher calling of martyrdom cannot, in all good conscience, go on to seek excusal from their chosen suffering. They risk allegations of insincerity if they do. Jesus did not have a break from the cross. If it is too much to bear, the selfless employee needs to reconsider their choice, as the soaring resignation rate in the Met suggests that many are doing.

Resignation and job change is, within reason, a feature of dynamic economies and a way for people who are unhappy in their work to try something different. But it is in danger of becoming a thing of the past. A 2012 PwC report on global trends in 'human capital' found that, whereas 15% of employees in the Asia-Pacific region resigned their position in any given year, only 9% of UK employees did the same.[4] The trend, in terms of the stagnancy of the labour market in the West, is downwards. PwC's 2014 report found that, whereas more than 10% of Western European employees resigned their role in 2007, this had halved to approximately 5% by 2013.[5]

Employment is a relationship freely entered into, not a gulag or an arranged marriage, although we increasingly seem to view as a disaster people's decision to leave a job with which they cannot cope, or which is making them unhappy. The Stevenson/Farmer report 'Thriving at Work' is a good example of this error of thinking.[6] It depicts the turnover within the labour market of people who consider themselves to have a mental health problem as always being a bad thing. Yet some degree of fluidity within the labour market is healthy. It provides dating opportunities for job-seekers and prospective employers. This is the way they can give feedback to each about how they are perceived, how they might make themselves more attractive, and what kind of partner seems to suit them best.

For their part, the employer needs to come off the fence and make decisions. Are expectations for the employee's role reasonable, and have they provided what support they can? If the answer to both questions is 'yes', then by extension the problem is with the employee, who, if they are incapable, will need to be managed through the capability route. As proponents of wellbeing, is the employer then going to prioritise the business need to manage the incapability over the employee's welfare, which, in the short term at least, will predictably suffer from the process? The employee's welfare may sometimes—much as no-one wants to say it—be secondary to the needs of the organisation.

What is the alternative in such a situation? Some would urge the employer to make 'wellbeing' interventions such as additional rest breaks, flexible working or mindfulness sessions on the grounds that these can improve employee productivity, and so serve a business need in themselves. This is fair enough in the case of stressed but capable employees (see Chapter 21), but such interventions can only help the employee to realise their potential—not to exceed it. It is reminiscent of the old joke about the patient due to undergo hand surgery, who is reassured by his surgeon that he will be able to play the piano post-operatively. 'That is fantastic,' replies the patient. 'I never could before!' In the eyes of some employees failing in their role, and of managers desperate to avoid managing them, the concept of wellbeing can be stretched beyond absurdity. It may be taken to mean amending a role to match the capability of an individual incapable of the job the employer actually needs done. This is arguably more of a capitulation than a wellbeing intervention, and brings us back to the principle that employment is offered as a means to an end, and not as an end in itself.

Through medicalising what is in truth a relationship problem—albeit within a contractual relationship—the different parties hope to pursue their agendas surreptitiously and without the burden of responsibility for their own decisions. The employee may harbour the hope that a suitably paternalistic doctor will respond to their plea for help, and issue an edict to the employer as to how the role should be adapted. This spares the employee from having to negotiate a resolution to the problem themselves. Some managers, meanwhile, are so hopeless in motivating and policing their teams that they cling to the forlorn hope of a suitably Inquisition-like doctor acting on their behalf and mandating the individual's immediate return to work. The concept of drapetomania has been resurrected within these dysfunctional organisations. They see a doctor's prescription that the employee must return to their post as the only means by which they can legitimately restrain their slaves from fleeing, now that leg-irons and toe amputations would be beyond the pale.

The great epidemics of history such as smallpox and polio were generally brought to an end through a preventative approach, entailing vaccination with the infectious agents. Stress is an infectious meme that has taken hold, but there are ways of inoculating against it. When recruiting amongst the merchants of Venice, employers should make clear from the outset the true nature of the deal, which is one of reciprocity first and altruism second, rather than the other way around. Employees should be clear that they are entering a bond, and that if they do not deliver what has been promised then there will be a penalty. In particular, the employer will consistently enforce what has been agreed, irrespective of how much this may distress the individual. Where the employer funds initiatives intended to optimise employee health, they should contextualise these in terms of productivity rather than wellness. There should be no ambiguity about the cold fact that, much as the manager wishes the recruit to be happy and well during their career, this is subservient to their obligation to protect the interests of the organisation as a whole.

Employees should be dissuaded from casually entering unsuitable arrangements in the manner of Antonio. Then expectations would be better aligned with reality, and the scope for disaffection that much less. If the role involves regular receipt of abusive and unpleasant calls from aggrieved customers, then that is how it should be described, not as an opportunity for a bright and people-focussed individual to progress their career in a fast-paced environment. There is no formal educational requirement to become a police officer, but the starting salary is around £20,000, with a pay scale making £38,000 achievable within approximately seven years.[7] For those applicants who have not calculated that danger money is a component of their pay, it is important that this is made clear. Otherwise a career spent dealing with, and sometimes fighting, some of the most unpleasant members of society—often at 3 in the morning—is going to be one of perpetual disappointment and growing bitterness.

It does not follow that their managers can therefore behave in the manner of Shylock. For one thing, the most the manager can demand from the employee is their job, not their life. And employees are entitled to expect fair treatment. If the worker can propose alternative means of achieving the same objectives, and the manager can find no reasonable objection, then pragmatism should prevail. In all cases, whether or not the two parties can see eye to eye, civility and even kindness from management should be the order of the day—both of which are quite compatible with also being honest and consistent. If we returned to the basics of the employment contract—reminding employees that it is a condition of their continued employment that they honour the promises they have made, and managers of their duty to be reasonable and honest—we should see the stress epidemic recede into another footnote of history.

Currently we are pursuing an accelerant approach to the problem of stress, and remain busily occupied with heaping the funeral pyre underneath our economy. Wellness initiatives, counselling, psychology and indeed psychiatry are all very well for people who—if restored to health—have innate capability for the role in question. But when the fundamental problem is not a transient medical condition, but a mismatch between the needs of the role and the aptitude of the individual, it is a wholly different matter. Then, ill-conceived wellness initiatives provide the kindling, funded access to counselling, psychology and medical care provide the tinder, and any one of the countless perceived injustices amongst the modern workforce can provide the spark.

15

THE BLAME GAME

A small proportion of the working age population are unavoidably sick because their medical problems are simply insurmountable barriers to them working. Then there is a similarly small group of deliberately sick people, fraudsters, whose sickness is fabricated and who would be ensconced on the beaches of northern Spain irrespective of all the help and support that anyone could offer them, for as long as the fraud investigators had not caught up with them.

But the majority of sick people, perhaps anywhere between 50 and 75 per cent in my estimation, retain capacity for work. In the right circumstances and with the right support, they would be able to remain in the workplace, and everyone would be better off for them doing so. The endemic level of avoidable sickness in Britain today is an indictment. It reflects the dearth of practical advice and support for people who are struggling to stay in work but nevertheless sliding slowly towards the door for health-related reasons.

Of all the people who are in a position to intervene, it is generally the manager who has the most power, and the most to gain if they are successful in stabilising the person in work. They are likely to spend as much of the waking day with the individual as their partner or spouse, if not more, so they are well placed to know when all is not well and to have some inkling as to why that might be. In terms of then doing something about it, even first line managers have at least some degree of control over the workplace. Maintaining someone in work might require some temporary additional effort for the busy supervisor, such as a reassuring catch-up call every few days or some rerostering. Even so, this is less arduous than having to make time-consuming and costly arrangements for the employee's work to be covered in the event that they go sick. Yet managers tend to be conspicuous by their absence as the slow car crash of imminent sickness absence plays out. Why do they prefer to lie low?

Dealing with people can be tiring and difficult. Not everyone is a people person, and even people people can have their fill sometimes. The enforced politeness and euphemisms that characterise industrial relations, with a plethora of employment law discouraging honesty and directness, is especially wearisome. When the employee is ill and the news that the manager has to impart is not welcome—that the employee's attendance or performance is unsustainable, or their conduct unacceptable—this makes conversation particularly hazardous for the demoralised manager. No-one wants to stand accused of heartlessness, or to find themselves being mobbed by angry colleagues. And with a progressively medicalised workforce, the probability of an absent, underperforming or poorly behaving employee having a diagnosis to brandish as a medical shield is high. If the employee's behaviour has been especially dramatic—displays of histrionic emotion, public declarations of suicidal intent[i]—the reticence of the manager to have a conversation

---

[i] At least several times a week, I speak to managers distressed at hav-

about anything other than the weather and last night's television is palpable and understandable.

Confidence and morale amongst the management cadre will be further weakened if they themselves are poorly led. This problem is most acute in organisations with rambling and ungainly organograms that make decisive, coherent management action practically impossible. Sometimes the complexity is in a vertical sense, as with hierarchical organisations with a tall management pyramid consisting of multiple layers. In these institutions, there are incremental increases in responsibility between each successive grade. Promotions tending to be given according to the Peter principle,[ii] recipients of these new responsibilities have quite possibly been appointed just beyond their level of competence. The overall effect is of one slightly deficient tier atop another, rather like an ornate but sloppily made wedding cake. Alternatively, in flatter organisations, the hotchpotch of slightly overlapping management roles may sprawl horizontally with about as much clarity and definition as a Jackson Pollock drip painting.

You have to wonder why the employees of such organisations would venture to break from the ranks of the workers and into

---

ing had to deal with an employee threatening suicide after a conversation about their performance or conduct: for example their attendance, timekeeping, performance, behaviour towards colleagues or use of the company credit card.

[ii] Laurence Peter espoused his management theory of the Peter principle in his book of the same name, published in 1969. He reasoned that, when candidates are being selected for promotion, this is on the basis of their track record in their roles to date, not their capability in the role they have yet to attempt. On that basis, it follows that their ascent through the management chain stops only once their performance in their existing role is already inadequate: hence Peter's aphorism that 'managers rise to the level of their incompetence'.

the management chain. Rarely can it be because of a sadomasochistic enjoyment of office politics. Often it will be out of ambition to achieve personal and professional development. Those with the intellectual capacity to take a higher-level view of what is happening in their workplace have a natural desire to be more involved in reconfiguring the trainset rather than endlessly shunting the trucks. If they are 'people people' to any extent, if they have earnt the respect of those reporting to them by demonstrating technical competence across the roles they are managing, and if it is apparent that their motivation is the healthy one of wishing to see a job well done, then this is a very good start.

The spur for others to become managers may be less wholesome. A minority are simply unpleasant characters who derive enjoyment from exercising control over others. That said, the suggestion that anywhere between 3 and 20 per cent of them are psychopaths who happen to have made it into the boardroom rather than into prison, as some researchers claim, is perhaps leaning towards hyperbole.[1] More often, the lure of a management role is not so much power as money.

There is nothing inherently immoral or improper about taking on a bigger job for more money. Ambitious applicants can make perfectly competent and energised managers, provided that there are at least some edifying reasons why they are seeking promotion as well as pecuniary ones. The problem however—especially in vertiginous corporate structures with a parallel series of overlapping pay grades—is that the pay increment being offered may be too small. Just enough to tempt candidates seeking a slightly fancier set of letters on the boot-lid of their car, but not quite enough to sustain them through the relentless series of minicrises that they will have to negotiate amongst their team on a daily basis.

Often there is so little to differentiate these marginally better paid managers from their subordinates that it is unsurprising if their response to awkward situations is to look the other way. They may well live in the same streets, let alone the same towns, have children in the same class at the same schools, and drink in the same pubs. These managers, in name only, fear the hostility and reprisals of their peers more than the criticism of their own managers higher up the ranks. It was the prisoner-turned-guard kapos of the concentration camps, paid meagre privileges to supervise the other inmates, who were the most despised. Similarly, junior managers often attract the contempt of their reports in a way, paradoxically, that more senior management does not. Downtrodden employees expect no favours from the top brass. The latter are remote, not people they identify with to any extent, and callous tyranny is deemed to be in their nature. But the kapo manager—someone like them who should know better—is guilty of the twin crimes of oppression and treason to boot.

The obvious solution that some teams of employees adopt in the face of this conundrum—everyone wanting a little more pay, none wanting to manage—was brought home to me by a civil servant. She was locked in an upsetting interpersonal dispute with a colleague whom she believed to be a bully, and explained that she lacked any confidence that her manager would intervene because he was 'coming to the end of his turn'. Of the five employees in the team, every single one had managed the other four for some length of time in the preceding years, until the heat had become too much for them, it was time to request a demotion, and the baton was passed to another team member. In this way, all could fairly share the miserly manager's increment, but none would be expected to actually manage anything. On each occasion that the glaring deficiencies of local line management became too much for senior management to bear, the kaleidoscope would be reshaken by the manager's resignation and acceptance of a demoted role—just prior to the instigation of a development plan—and the process could begin again.

Management according to Buggins' turn is a glorious example of the human capacity for ingenuity and adaptability to any set of circumstances. It does mean, however, that behaviours exhibited within the workplace begin to resemble *Lord of the Flies* more than a human resources training manual. The notion that kapo managers will decisively manage their peers, for perhaps a few hundred or thousand pounds more a year, is delusional—but it is one that senior management often maintains. Many managers are managers because they have demonstrated technical competence in their field, and not by virtue of their emotional intelligence. Yet they end up in a position where they are managing people, not equipment or process flows. The support they receive in learning skills that are new and not necessarily innate is patchy at best. When it comes to learning how to manage people who are ill and flagging in their efforts to remain in work, managers receive very little helpful or practical training.

When a ship's captain, even an experienced captain, is having to navigate the waters of a difficult port that they rarely visit, it is the norm for a pilot—with good local knowledge of the dangers, and of the safest ways around them—to come aboard. Similarly, within large organisations it was once common practice for the human resources team to offer more intensive support and advice to managers at times when they were in unfamiliar waters, such as when dealing with employees who may be ill, sick or alleging injury to feelings arising from their work. In the post-recessionary years, this trend has begun to reverse amid talk of wanting to empower managers. This is empowerment in the sense of 'You're on your own!' Of course the true driver is financial, in the absence of any inexplicable uptick in the competence of the management chain to deal with these issues alone. In hard times, the port authority withdraws the pilots, and the captains are alone in their wheelhouses. Poorly skilled, inexperienced and unsupported managers are left to their own devices when confronted with the problem of managing someone who is finding it increasingly difficult to cope. Worse, as if sailing blind in treacherous waters weren't bad enough, they receive conflicting orders from senior command as to what they should be doing—from those not actually in the engine room, but swanning about up top, yet considering themselves an expert.

Those managers incentivised by a bonus to achieve outcome targets want the first line manager to achieve these at all costs. Meanwhile, the legal team, and health and safety, will circulate horror stories from the employment tribunal—perhaps even the inquest—that were caused by the bungling of other managers. For them, the avoidance of all risk is paramount. The finance bean-counters will have their own cost-cutting agenda, and it will be neither operational nor safety-oriented. Amidst this chaos, human resources—perhaps even a self-styled 'wellness champion', in an organisation sufficiently engorged to justify such a role—will periodically cascade training too. This is to the effect that the manager should be doing more to ensure the joie de vivre, thinness, fitness and overall attractiveness of their team.

Whether the line manager operates in an overly tall organisation or an overly fat one, and whether they are a permanent fixture or merely keeping the seat warm, the experience of being at the bottom of a disorderly management chain is one of confusion and miscommunication. When disaster inevitably strikes, and blame is being apportioned from the life rafts, they learn from the scapegoating of colleagues who tried to adhere to one or other of the conflicting commands. The safest option is to stay well away from the controls. As a result, the ship is doomed to collision sooner or later, but line managers can at least be sure not to have left any fingerprints at the accident scene.

It is little wonder that poleaxed inaction is commonly the default mode of junior management in situations that are anything other than the plain sailing of business as usual. In the words of one middle-grade civil servant I encountered early in my occupational medicine career, who had three decades of service behind him and six months of full-paid 'stress leave' to look forward to before collecting his pension, 'No-one here ever got sacked for doing nothing. You only ever get sacked for doing something, and it turning out wrong.'

The line manager lacking any confidence in dealing with a tricky management issue desperately needs a justification for it to become someone else's problem. To whom can they lob the sizzling bomb to be defused, or at least in someone else's hands when it blows up? In a hypermedicalised society such as ours, with a little imagination most dilemmas can be portrayed as medical in some contrived way or other. In organisations with access to occupational health services, it is the occupational physician who is generally the sucker, left holding the unwelcome present when the fuse wire has fizzled away. What ruse might the resourceful manager use to facilitate the transfer?

Their fairly transparent tactic is the parlour game of 'I'm Not a Doctor'. It is not to be found formally recorded in any management manual, but is a secret spell handed down from one generation of managers to the next, and as useful to them as anything Harry Potter might have learnt at Hogwarts. By incanting this phrase in response to a stressed employee who ostensibly has a health problem, all normal management responsibility for that individual is magically alleviated. Thus, at least in the mind of the manager, the requirement to engage with people who may be emotional, awkward or even aggressive is avoided once they can be shoehorned into the role of the patient. Managers can be as keen to medicalise the employee's problems as the person themselves. The commonest variant of this game arises when the employee is underperforming or behaving in ways that are unacceptable, and the line manager is especially reluctant to draw this to their attention. This may be because, the last time anyone attempted to benchmark the employee's performance against management's and not their own expectations, it resulted in a scene, threats of suicide, a grievance, or a lengthy period of absence—or, for the most traumatised managers, all four.

Sometimes the willingness to play I'm Not a Doctor is not for fear of upsetting the employee but out of concern at the possible reaction of colleagues if it is the manager who is seen to wield the knife. These managers, like Lady Macbeth, hope that someone else will do their dirty work. This is especially common amongst more militant, unionised workforces where mobbing behaviours are seen, and when the line manager is a kapo manager, perceived by the workforce as only being management in a technical sense. The lack of respect for their authority means that these managers fear reprisals in response to any unpopular action they might take, like an elder child left in charge and secretly hoping for the parents' return to rein in the more rowdy siblings.

Alternatively, it may not be the employee or the team that the manager fears so much as their own conscience. Sometimes it is obvious to all that an employee's capability is grossly impaired by serious illness, but no-one wants to say it. This is especially true with progressive neurological disorders such as multiple sclerosis, whose sufferers' deterioration is often gradual and painfully apparent. Although the unfortunate truth may be that this is intolerable for the organisation, the manager finds it impossible to break this bad news, because doing so would jar so greatly with their self-identity as a Nice Person. Much kinder, they reason, for the employee to be told by someone they have probably never met before and may well never see again, and who is in no position to know how well they perform in practice. Thus the employee is sent to see this medical hitman, or hitwoman, under the disingenuous guise of receiving medical support rather than the last rites for their employment. Assuming that I'm Not a Doctor pans out in the way that managers hope, they begin preparing for a round of My Hands Are Tied, and perhaps some crocodile tears for good measure.

The predictable denouement of I'm Not a Doctor, though, is disappointing for the manager. Unsurprisingly, doctors tend not to enjoy telling people that they are no longer able to do their job to someone else's satisfaction, on that someone else's behalf. If they are to be the bearer of bad news, they would quite appreciate some evidence that what they are saying—which they know will result in the employee's dismissal—is actually the case.

Conventionally, the first and most obvious person from whom to seek such evidence would be the line manager. They have the advantage of a good technical understanding of the role and its objectives, and spend around eight hours per day with the individual in the workplace to watch how, in practice, they perform against these. More to the point, one of the core functions that justifies the manager's wage increment is to be responsible for appraising capability. For the seriously underperforming employee, the personnel file should, in theory, catalogue a series of informal and subsequently formal management interventions designed to bring the problem to the individual's attention and to try and help them to perform better.

But given the premise of I'm Not a Doctor—the strange assumption that, because the manager lacks training in detection and treatment of disease, they are unable to appraise capability—no useful information will be forthcoming from that quarter. Whatever entries were made in the personnel file to evidence management's concerns were made in magic ink, which the manager nevertheless expects the medical advisor to be able to read. Instead the doctor must turn to the individual to ask them how they feel they manage in their job. Turkeys, though, do not vote for Christmas. Most people who are in fear of losing their employment will tend to answer leading questions about their capability with 'not too bad, thank you doctor'.

When the medical advisor reports to the manager that they consider the individual to be fit, since neither the employer nor the employee has identified any problems with their performance, this will be met with righteous indignation. Managers who play I'm Not a Doctor are firm devotees of the medical model and assume that a medical degree confers extraordinary powers of perception, because this is a convenient belief system for them. The practitioner who does not say what the manager sees as being patently obvious—but are too scared to say themselves—must therefore be a buffoon of the first order. The reality is that ill people are not malfunctioning robots. Testing their circuitry, as doctors do when they chat to them and ask them to wiggle their limbs, is really very poorly predictive of how they actually function in the workplace.

In the face of obvious and severe disability, the doctor can say little to an employee adamant that they are nevertheless coping in their role, except that this is surprising and commendable. Rarely can they be so sure of their ground as to accuse the employee of fibbing. In any case, how are they to know how lenient the manager is prepared to be about their performance? Contractually, it is not the doctor who is buying the services of the individual. Only the person who is—the employer, in the form of the manager—can decide what they expect in return for their money. This is particularly so given the legal requirement for employers to make reasonable adjustments—which might include some reduction in normal productivity or performance targets for a role—for disabled workers.

Whether you are well or ill, in most cases it is your manager who decides how satisfactory your performance is. The etiquette of employment is that it is also courteous of them to tell you directly rather than via their medical emissaries. The only exception to this rule is when the employee is working in a safety-critical role[iii] and where there is a medical condition with the potential to prevent them from working safely. Examples include the risk of sudden incapacitation in a patient susceptible to seizures, or paroxysmal abnormal cardiac rhythms that suddenly reduce the pumping efficiency of their heart. Then, medical expertise may be invaluable in making a careful assessment of the medical risk. Sometimes it will be the unhappy but necessary duty of the occupational physician to have to advise that the individual is 'unfit' to operate the crane, drive the forklift or direct the air traffic—irrespective of how the person might feel or indeed perform on a day-to-day basis.

In today's service economy, however, only a minority of jobs are safety-critical in nature, and only a small subset of the people working in them will have any illness that seriously compromises their safety. Most of the time, for most people, whether or not they can do their job has little to do with medical risk (where the doctor is the expert) and everything to do with capability (where the manager is). Medical expertise will help the doctor advise whether an employee's incapability or poor behaviour might have a medical basis, when this is not otherwise obvious; whether it is likely to be a temporary or permanent problem; and what could be done to assist the situation. It will not help them to appraise the employee's worth to their employer in pounds and pence.

Despite this, we still persist in talking about 'fitness for work' and maintaining the pretence that this is something that is

---

[iii] A role where, if the employee were impaired by symptoms of whatever kind whilst performing their work, there would be a risk of substantial harm. This might be harm to the individual (as with a roofer susceptible to blackouts), to other people (as with a narcoleptic railway signaller) or to both (as with an airline pilot incapacitated by a heart attack).

assessed effectively by doctors. In essence, the act of sickness certification itself—outside of a safety-critical environment—is an institutionalised version of I'm Not a Doctor.

16

SELF-HELP

The health and safety approach—trying to prevent injuries and illness in the first place, providing medical care when these attempts fail—has been enormously successful.

The impressive achievements of healthcare in the 350 years since Thomas Sydenham's *Observationes mediciae* have already been described. As for safety, when it comes to the hard endpoints of death or serious injuries, such as fractures and dislocations, work is safer than it has ever been. In the forty years that followed the introduction of the 1974 Health and Safety at Work Act, the number of fatal workplace injuries in the UK fell by about 85 per cent. Non-fatal injuries—at least, those reported to the Health and Safety Executive—fell by 77 per cent.[1]

In large part this is because the number of jobs that are inherently dangerous has dwindled as the economy has evolved. Within a couple of generations, we transformed from a primarily industrial nation of miners and factory workers to a service sector economy of office workers, hairdressers, baristas and nail-bar technicians. In 1950 the coal industry employed 691,000 people; by 2004 that figure was 6,000.[2] The size of the UK hair and beauty industry was estimated at 245,795 workers in 2012.[3] What dirty and dangerous jobs do still need to be done are largely done by machine. Alternatively—sad but true—they have been exported to countries with lower standards of health and safety legislation, by multinational corporates that would prefer to have the work done cheaply rather than safely.[4]

But it is not all down to technology, automation and globalisation. Health and safety legislation can take much of the credit too. During the nineteenth century, it developed on a reactive, piecemeal basis. It sequentially addressed particular hazards in the mines and factories that had especially offended the national conscience thanks to the pamphleteers of the period.[i] In the latter part of the twentieth century, it matured into an all-encompassing, preventative philosophy. As living standards improved over time, so we became less accepting of risk associated with employment. Employers are now legally obliged to deliberately envisage the dangers of the tasks performed by their employees (risk assessment) through legislation such as the Health and Safety at Work Regulations 1999. Where harm can be foreseen, they have a duty to implement whatever measures are necessary to reduce the risk to a level that is 'as low as reasonably practicable'. There is the potential for criminal prosecution and imprisonment of managers or boards who fail in their duty of care to safeguard employees, through instruments such as the Corporate Manslaughter and Corporate Homicide Act 2007.

The dramatic fall in workplace fatalities over a relatively short period shows that the safety approach—requiring employers to be proactive in identifying and managing risks, and prosecuting and jailing those who don't—clearly works. But, despite making work

---

[i] Such as the Cotton Mills and Factories Act 1819, which prohibited the employment of children until they had reached the ripe old age of 9.

safer, the health and safety paradigm has certainly not resulted in fewer people being sick from their work—and might even have contributed to that problem. Rates of sickness rose steadily during the latter twentieth century and have only receded a little in the twenty-first, despite workplaces becoming much safer and healthcare much more effective. The problem is that the safety approach, just like the medical approach, has its limits. And, just like medicine, when safety is stretched beyond the limits of its usefulness, it becomes useless, and even counterproductive.

The safety approach is useful when there is an unarguable relationship between a cause and an effect, and when the effect is serious. Take the perennial problem of young, biddable apprentices periodically falling from great heights through fragile ceilings or from rickety, jury-rigged scaffolds, thanks to the miserliness of their unscrupulous employers in failing to provide appropriate equipment. The association between falling 40 feet and immediately afterwards having a depressed skull fracture, an acquired brain injury, long bone fractures or a flail chest, or indeed being dead, is self-evident. The effects are undeniably grave. It is this kind of tragedy, major injuries sustained in high-hazard environments, that safety legislation has been so effective at addressing. Sadly, such incidents still happen—but much less than was once the case. There are still plenty of cowboys, but they are more likely to behave responsibly, even if this is out of a healthy fear of fines and jail time rather than genuine concern for those they employ.

But as the strength of the causal association, and the severity of the injury, begins to lessen, so the safety approach has less and less to offer. Today, many allegedly workplace-related 'injuries' are so subtle that they are impossible to see, and the association with the workplace is more tenuous. Aching backs, aching arms and bruised egos are all very common anyway. Whilst the rise of reports of back pain in particular is attributed to the prevalence of sedentary desk jobs, this explanation ignores the decline of equally back-breaking manufacturing jobs. In this landscape, the safety approach can achieve more harm than good. Naive efforts to 'educate' and raise awareness, catastrophisation, hysteria and the potential for compensation or preferential treatment from the employer can all mean that the rates of these more minor problems begin to rise rather than fall. Over the generations, different conditions that meet these criteria of hazy existence and even hazier causation have followed a signature pattern of emergence, explosion and subsequent decline. Society cottons on and tires of them sooner or later. Then they recede, in readiness for the next 'useful illness'.[ii] This has been the pattern of the epidemics of industrial low back pain and repetitive strain 'injury'. The current stress epidemic will one day be added to the list.

It is as though, at any point in history, there is a proportion of the workforce ready and waiting for the next health and safety scare. Some will be disgruntled and seeking, consciously or subconsciously, a means of symbolising the hurt they feel at the hand of their employer, and of achieving the more considerate treatment they feel is their due. Being diagnosed as the victim of a work-caused injury is an effective means of achieving both. Others are schemers, waiting for the next scam. And still more are simply suggestible, prone to believing health scares and becoming swept up in the frenzy.

The waxing and waning of these epidemics should be no surprise. They are further proof—if proof were needed—that sickness is predominantly a sociological phenomenon. It is driven by people's attitudes, beliefs and economic circumstances, much more so than by their biology or injury rate. Predictably, measures which have undoubtedly been successful in treating serious diseases and avoiding serious accidents have had little impact on sickness levels.

[ii] See Malleson's *Whiplash and other useful illnesses*.

Managers lack confidence in dealing with health issues and so they cling to the health and safety approach as a comfort blanket. But most of the problems that their staff experience, whether they are notionally 'health' issues or 'safety' ones, would in truth be better managed in-house and without making such a fuss. There are employees whose backs or necks or arms ache, in common with the way most people's backs and necks and arms ache from time to time. Or people who are grieving, or worried about a sick relative, or not coping well with their work, or struggling with relationship breakdowns, or who have fallen out with colleagues, as sometimes happens to everybody else. These are people who need empathy and practical advice and support, rather than being propelled into the clutches of external experts, which will only ratchet the tension up a notch. It isn't just patients who can be hypochondriacal: organisations can be too. Western companies—employees and their managers—need to rethink what it means to be ill and to develop a greater capacity for self-managing minor health problems within the organisation, rather than outsourcing to clinicians.

In *The Last Well Person*, Nortin Hadler explains that being well does not mean the absence of symptoms, but retaining a sense of invincibility despite their presence, and not paying undue heed to them. Sometimes the person's symptoms are sufficiently different, severe or sinister[iii] that their confidence in their ability to self-manage is shaken. On those occasions, entirely appropri-

---

[iii] An individual's ability to recognise symptoms that, whilst not unbearable, may warrant prompt consultation with a doctor depends on their exposure to disease awareness campaigns and their knowledge about the 'sentinel' symptoms of serious disease. This imparts an understanding of the significance of coughing blood in phlegm as a predictor of lung cancer, or of passing blood in urine as a predictor of genitourinary cancer.

ately, they seek healthcare and, sometimes, there will be a serious underlying medical problem meaning that they should become patients. Often there will not be; explanation and reassurance is all that is needed to restore their autonomy as a person coping with the challenges of life, whether physical symptoms such as backache and migraines, or psychological ones such as anxiety or low mood.

Clearly, sometimes illness is exclusively defined by biological factors—disease—entirely beyond the control of the individual. There is no need to go looking for any ulterior explanation as to why such people are seeking healthcare. In the acute phase, when they need emergency treatment, trying to place their symptoms in a wider psychological and social context might be a dangerous distraction. The patient who wakes at 3am clutching their chest, experiencing the worst pain they have ever felt and with a morbid fear of dying there and then,[iv] does not need extensive psychoanalysis, but instead to be conveyed to the cardiac catheter suite of the nearest district general hospital without delay.

Most instances of illness, though, are less dramatic, urgent or clear-cut. Much of the time the symptoms experienced by the individual are not so very different to those being felt by many others.[5] They feel the need to seek healthcare when their coping mechanisms have been overwhelmed, perhaps because—at the best of times—their capacity to cope is simply less than that of other people, or maybe because of other worrying and distressing circumstances in their lives that are also wearing them down. Frequently the conversion of person to patient is driven more by social factors and their individual propensity to seek healthcare than by the severity of their symptoms.

[iv] The *angor animi*, a belief that one is dying, often experienced by the heart attack victim.

It follows that medicine—most effective in the treatment of disease, rather than in addressing the unpleasant experiences that afflict us all from time to time—is largely unhelpful to many patients. The medicalisation of their problems can be positively detrimental. Then, the patient has to contend with the side-effects of unnecessary treatments and, as they develop dependent relationships with those treating them, their confidence in their ability to manage their own lives—their sense of their own invincibility—begins to ebb away.

It also disenfranchises those around them from feeling able to help. When problems are presented in a human context, other human beings feel able to respond in kind. 'I am so frustrated that I was not selected for promotion' is met with 'I can understand that; maybe it wasn't for you this time around?' The response to 'I feel sad at my partner's cheating' might be 'I don't blame you. If that is how they treat the important people in their life maybe you are better off with without them?' When one person complains, 'My back aches when I have been sat for too long,' another might reply, 'So does mine! I get up and move around every twenty minutes or so.'

When the same issues are presented in medical form—'I have a diagnosed adjustment disorder'; 'I am depressed'—or perhaps even Latinised for full effect—'I have moderately severe lumbosacral spondyloarthritis'—those around them with an unhealthy respect for medicine are rendered mute in their humility. Medicalisation of life's problems denudes the great majority of people who are not healthcare professionals of the ability to apply their own life experience, or the soft skills of common sense and emotional intelligence, for the benefit of others. The great shame is that this is often exactly the kind of help most needed by the person, and that which they are least likely to receive in a healthcare setting. The prevailing dogma that, when someone is experiencing symptoms, it is solely professionals who are in a position to help has a stultifying effect on the capacity of people to care for one another.[v]

In real life people have mildly unpleasant experiences—symptoms—much of the time, and amateur rather than professional help is exactly what is needed. Often the onset of symptoms is for no discernible reason; in a similarly mysterious way they will pass of their own accord, and there is little effective treatment in the meantime. When the person feels confident in their ability to cope, then such temporary unpleasantness does not discombobulate them. They are copers, and with the morale-boosting support and encouragement of those around them—including their managers—they will cope with this too.

'This' might be a week of backache, or a suddenly tender wrist, or a day of inexplicably feeling blue, or a temporary crisis of confidence. It might be specifically rooted worries, for the health of a frail parent, the looming exams of a child, or the unusually frequent business trips of a partner. None of these are things that will be helped by sowing seeds of anxiety in the person's mind that they herald something worse medically, or by pretending that there is any quick fix either. They are all things that are made easier to bear with the acknowledgement of others, a kind word, and reassurance and encouragement that, whatever happens, things will probably be okay.

Very often, when an employee is experiencing all but the most severe symptoms, they could cope with their work—perhaps modified slightly, so as to reduce or avoid those tasks that they find difficult or uncomfortable at that point in time—with a little reassurance and empathy from those around them. This might require a conversation with their manager, as simple as agreeing

---

[v] What Illich described as cultural and social iatrogenesis: the harms caused by healers (see Chapter 10, fn xvii).

that—if the individual's back is aching that week and they would struggle to sustain their ten-hour shift—they might work a six-hour shift until feeling better, if they feel they could manage that instead. Or, it may be that the person's panic attacks are worse than normal and fears of embarrassment or of being trapped in work are beginning to put them off attending. In this case, they may simply need the reassurance that no-one will mind if they do disappear for a few minutes at short notice in order to have a break somewhere private.

Unfortunately, mythical beliefs about the perils of work and the virtues of rest remain commonplace, and act as a barrier to these kinds of conversations. Many managers feel that talking to people who are not '100 per cent well' about the circumstances in which they would feel able to continue working would be tantamount to cruelty, rather than an attempt at helping them.

This myth that it is unwise to be in work if one is less than 100 per cent fit—as though anyone is 100 per cent fit most of the time—helps to push ill people out of the workplace and into sickness.[vi] The idea that work is inherently dangerous, and that people need to be fully on their toes in order to survive it, persists as a subliminal anxiety in our cultural DNA. It may have its roots in the Industrial Revolution, which introduced perilous, unguarded

---

[vi] This kind of attitude is still encountered. In the biopsychosocial framework, when it is apparent during a consultation with an employee, it constitutes a 'yellow flag' (relating to unhelpful health beliefs that can act as needless barriers to work). Sometimes it is evident in referrals received from managers seeking reassurance that the employee 'is 100% fit', with the insinuation that they should not attend work otherwise. In 2015 Professor Kim Burton and his team prepared an excellent 'line manager's toolbox' for the Health and Safety Executive ('Research Report 1053'), which referred to the fact that such myths still exist in our culture and that dispelling them is an important part of optimising people's ability to work.

machinery that periodically claimed life and limb in a way that would have been alien to those previously used to the backbreaking—but unmechanised—work of subsistence agriculture. It was entirely rational and healthy to fear the risks of working with steam hammers, power looms and Blake's 'Satanic Mills', but as the world of work has transformed, these unadapted anxieties have become unhelpful. The worst dangers facing the average mollycoddled office worker of today are paper cuts, broken air conditioning and fingers trapped in errant filing cabinets.

The related myth of rest as a panacea, also a prevalent and unhelpful belief, helps to pull ill people out of work. It seems to have its origins in the Victorian era, the chief culprit being the American physician Silas Weir Mitchell. His 'rest cure'—which entailed confinement to bed for weeks on end—gained currency as treatment for the neurasthenia (PTSD) of Civil War veterans, and for nervous disorders and hysteria. Whilst a superficially appealing idea to the modern worried well, it must have been dispiritingly tedious for those who actually experienced it. That is quite apart from the risks of venous thromboembolism, pneumonia and bone demineralisation that we would be concerned about today for even relatively short periods of enforced bed rest.

Understandably, those subjected to this treatment complained bitterly about it. It was Weir's achievement to enrage not one but two vociferous female novelists of the Victorian era. Virginia Woolf was a patient who went on to ridicule Weir's methods in *Mrs Dalloway*. Charlotte Perkins Gilman's semiautobiographical short story *The Yellow Wallpaper* centred on her experience of the rest cure whilst being treated by Weir Mitchell for postpartum psychosis. But despite the astute warnings of these wise women, both with far more sense than their doctor, the rest cure captured the Victorian imagination. It had a certain appeal at a time when much illness was mistakenly believed to be the result of exhausted nerve cells or, in women, to be 'hysterical' in origin, the result of some presumed ovular or uterine hormonal hyperactivity.

In fact our brain cells cannot be likened to batteries, nor is the female reproductive system the root cause of all female illness. The evidence is that Weir Mitchell got it wrong: being able to keep working whilst ill, not resting, is therapeutic in most cases. People's symptoms tend to be less severe, and to resolve more quickly, when they are able to continue working to some degree. The irony of sickness in post-industrial societies is that the principal reasons why people fall out of work—common mental health problems, back pain, arm pain—are all things that are generally exacerbated, rather than helped, by being inactive. Maintaining normal life as far as possible, including the routine, distraction and sociability of work, is often the best medicine.[6]

When managers are enlightened about the therapeutic value of work, and are not hamstrung by paranoid fears that work is going to make matters worse, direct engagement with the employee about the ways they could be helped to keep working has many benefits. For one thing, it is more efficient than paying for medical opinion in situations where it is common sense and pragmatism that is needed. The advice that occupational health professionals give to managers is boringly predictable because, normally, what would help the employee is self-evident from the nature of their symptoms. Someone who finds it painful to sit for more than thirty minutes might be encouraged to stand up and walk around more regularly than that; someone very tired might need shorter shifts until they have regained their stamina.

Any manager who has referred more than a few employees with back pain will already know when referring the next one what the advice will be. The more they are able to regularly alter their posture, to avoid awkward or extreme movements of their spine, and to refrain from lifting heavy items as far as they can, the more comfortable they are likely to be and the more likely they are to be able to remain in work. It is no good an employer bemoaning the monotonous similarity of the advice given by medical advisors, as if their suggestions should be varied solely to keep things interesting, if the referrals themselves are monotonously similar. Until an organisation develops the capacity to self-manage the more humdrum, commonplace problems which are part and parcel of human life, and learns that these are not a cause to hit the panic button, they are going to keep getting the same answers from their medical advisors.

Unfortunately, coughs, colds and tummy upsets are periodically a feature of normal life and there is rarely any point troubling one's doctor about them. Those that do cannot complain, when told to take paracetamol and plenty of fluids, that this is the same advice they were given the last time they made an unnecessary visit to the surgery. It is just the same for needy employers who refer every employee at the first twinge of backache or at their first report of stress.

It makes immediate financial sense for managers to ask employees who are temporarily unwell with these low-key health issues about the adjustments they feel would be helpful in their work, rather than asking an occupational health professional to do the same, transcribe the response and relay it to them. The individual is uniquely able to know how their symptoms affect their day-to-day function, the things that tend to help, and the things that make matters worse. They also have first-hand experience of all the component tasks of their job. The money that has been saved from making an unnecessary occupational health referral, consisting of questions with self-evident answers, can be used to offset the cost of the adjustment that the medical advisor will certainly recommend anyway.

More than that, keeping things in the family makes business sense too. It will improve the quality of the line manager relationship: something that will have a lasting pay-off in terms of greater engagement, motivation and goodwill. Imagine a relationship where your partner was struggling and seeking your support. If your response was to hand them the number of a counselling service then, whilst you may have saved yourself some time, it wouldn't be too long before you would need to start stocking up on microwave meals for one. Similarly, although an employer may think of an occupational health referral as a demonstration of care, it is easy to see how the employee might perceive it differently—and negatively. For example, they may interpret it as implying that they are not trusted, or considered sensible enough to know what will help them best. For the employee, to be listened to is to be believed and valued.

Often the manager may not quite be able to accommodate the individual in the way that they would ideally prefer. However, the employee is still more likely to endure what persisting symptoms they do have if they are persuaded that, nevertheless, the manager has tried their best and has at least done something. The human capital of the relationship is growing and the person's ability to cope is being cultivated. The illness becomes a shared enemy, not a stick with which the employee feels they need to beat the manager in order to gain their consideration. This is why the manager can so often be more influential over the course of the illness than the doctor. There is simply more that they can potentially do—so many ways in which they could potentially morph the role to better suit the employee's needs and thereby help to keep them in work. The doctor, on the other hand, is largely limited to watching and waiting for a common health problem to resolve of its own accord, in the absence of anything more useful they can do, which will be most of the time.[vii/7] The doctor holds a busted flush; it is the manager who is holding all the aces.

[vii] Voltaire's oft-repeated medical epigram was that the art of medicine consists of amusing the patient while nature cures the disease.

The penny is gradually dropping amongst enlightened employers that health issues within their organisations are managed best by managers engaging directly with their teams, not via medical avatars. As this realisation dawns, an inevitable question arises: how should managers, largely lacking in confidence, be helped to do this? This is normally contextualised with reference to the particular condition, especially mental health problems. How should a manager speak to someone who is stressed, as distinct from an employee who is anxious or depressed? Or someone who has been bereaved, or indeed who has fallen out with them? Sometimes the question will relate to serious, organic disease. How should they talk to someone with cancer, or multiple sclerosis, or Parkinson's disease? The very fact that these questions are asked is evidence of quite how dehumanised we have all become in a hypermedicalised society, stripped of our confidence in our ability to console, empathise with and support one another. It is as though we need a medical degree to be kind.

Managers love the notion of there being an algorithmic, procedural manual with which they can tackle any conceivable challenge they might encounter. Except at times when, in practice, they actually need to read the gargantuan tomes that result. Or when they have, unsurprisingly, managed to violate some sub-sub-subsection or other, and find themselves being metaphorically beaten about the head with the weighty policy document by a point-scoring union representative. But the idea of management by formula is self-defeating. Innumerable policies and clauses are generated by the infinite number of scenarios that can arise. If the new manager were actually to attempt to read them, they would be holding their retirement party before they had had time to actually manage anybody.

When a newly-diagnosed diabetic patient is being advised about the optimal self-management of their condition, they will be given dietary advice. This will include exhortation to eat more fruit, vegetables, wholegrains and dietary fibre, and to try and reduce the consumption of fat, sugar and salt. Their doctor is liable to describe this to them as a 'diabetic diet'. This is to the frustration of the dietitian. They will provide the correction that this is emphatically not a diabetic diet as such but a healthy one, the point being that it is particularly important for diabetic patients to eat healthily. So it is with the management of ill and sick employees. It is largely irrelevant what particular diagnosis the employee happens to have; there is one management style that is ideal for everyone, and that is good management. Ill employees are only different in that it is particularly important for them to receive good management, because they are less able to cope with poor management than other people.

I once reviewed the absence policy of an organisation, a single policy referring to multiple others, which itself ran to forty-eight pages. These bureaucratic monsters are some way from the brevity of Lincoln's Gettysburg address, and much less inspiring. Sometimes less is more. Policy is needed, but will only get you so far; beyond that, discretion, reasoning and intuition are needed. My experience is that the amount of policy an employer may have does not correlate especially well with how adroitly its managers handle sensitive issues. Rather, when things have gone wrong and the management has been poor, then typically it is because of a shortage of honesty, consistency, respect, kindness or care. This can be attributed to two factors, and both are in the employer's power to change: the degree of latitude afforded to managers, and their emotional intelligence in such situations, which can be improved through training. Fortunately, an emotionally intelligent approach to dealing with sick and ill people is substantially simpler than the more concrete thinkers amongst management may fear.

Honesty means giving employees the feedback that they need about their performance in the role, whether it is good or bad and whether the employee is well or ill. We all need this feed-back, whether it be for reassurance, as a warning to us that the relationship may be in danger if things don't improve, or—in the event that the situation is hopeless—as some warning of what is likely to follow, so that we can at least begin to prepare. Honest feedback is not a punishment. Whilst it may be difficult to hear, ignorance of reality can scarcely be better. It is perverse to give feedback freely to people who don't really need it and to with-hold it from the people who need it most. Yet withholding of information is a common response of managers dealing with ill employees, especially those with mental health problems, entirely contrary to the ethos of disability legislation—which is that dis-abled employees should not be disadvantaged—and for all the reasons that have already been rehearsed.

Consistency means not being coerced into saying something other than the truth in some effort to spare the pain of an employee struggling with the news of their incapability and the looming threat to their employment. False promises are incred-ibly tempting in the heat of the moment, whilst coaxing the employee down from the ledge, but are not kind in the long run, when they must be reneged upon. When an employee asks, 'I can't lose my job just because I'm ill, can I?', there is an easy answer and an honest one. There is nothing in employment law, or disability legislation, to preclude the dismissal of an ill employee on grounds of incapability, provided the employer has first ensured they have implemented what 'reasonable adjust-ments' they can in an effort to accommodate the disabled worker. The manager's choice, when positioned in this way, is between temporary gratification of the employee at the price of later bit-terness and resentment, and always being able to look the employee in the eye.

Consistency also means establishing and observing boundaries. It means that the manager cannot be confidant one day—a co-conspirator against the corporate machine (as David Brent might see himself)[viii]—and cold, performance-appraising terminator the next. Sadly, such is commercial life; managers need to take a position somewhere between these extremes. In a wider sense, consistency means that the same attitudes, behaviours and values are expected of people regardless of their seniority within the organisation—vital to a shared sense of organisational justice. I once took a call from a human resources business partner of a City firm. She admitted the litany of lecherous, abusive and bullying behaviours of a senior partner and lamented the extreme difficulty management now faced in knowing how to reintegrate him into the workplace. 'If it had been anyone else,' she reflected, seemingly oblivious as to how the firm had been hoist by its own petard in ever allowing things to get so far, 'he would have been long gone by now.'

In a medicalised world, respect for the individual, and their ability to make decisions for themselves, is too easily overlooked. We perceive someone who is ill as a patient first and a person second. The circumstances in which someone's mental state is so disturbed that they no longer have the capacity to make decisions for themselves are exceptionally few and far between, yet many employers seem to assume that this is true of anybody who brandishes a sick-note. Many of the conundrums created by employers, in their dealings with ill and sick people, are because they have forgotten the importance of dignifying the employee by respecting their ability to make their own decisions, and to face the consequences of doing so, just as everyone else does. Treating people like children, and wrapping them in cotton wool, has exactly the opposite effect to the one that is intended; it dis-

---

[viii] Perhaps the most often quoted of *The Office* protagonist's toe-curling management axioms, from the first episode of the first series, is 'I suppose I've created an atmosphere where I'm a friend first and a boss second. Probably an entertainer third.'

tresses and frustrates rather than soothes. For example, refraining from progressing an investigative or disciplinary process with the normal vigour will only leave the employee with it hanging over their head for longer.

Kindness and caring should not need further explanation—yet somehow, in this day and age, they do. They can take many forms but at their core is the recognition of another person's humanity and an outward demonstration, however subtle, of empathy and compassion for them. This may be practical, as with the manager who accompanies a sobbing employee to their medical appointment, dutifully waits for them,[ix] and helps them back home or back to work afterwards. It can be as seemingly trivial as momentary acknowledgment of the person in the midst of a hectic day. 'Seemingly' because that microsecond can matter to the person who is becoming ill and who feels that they are slipping out of sight.

Employment relationships are increasingly medicalised and legalised, but medical and legal approaches to life are not inherently kind or caring—they are clinical, technical and dehumanising. Likewise, the manager who insists on characterising every issue within their team solely in these terms, because they lack the soft skills to approach them as the human problems that they are, is not kind either. Organisational policies can go some way to improving the way in which managers can support their teams. Fundamentally, though, the single most important priority for any organisation wishing to decimate its sickness rates is simply training line managers to better appreciate the importance of treating their teams as human beings, rather than as diseased time-bombs or potential litigants.

[ix] Accompanying them to the consultation itself, as I have known some managers to do, strikes me as taking things to an unboundaried—and therefore inconsistent and unhelpful—extreme.

17

DEALING WITH REALITY

Something strange happens when a doctor is introduced as an intermediary in the relationship between an employee and their manager. As all alumni of the Hogwarts School of Management know, the manager loses all responsibility for managing the individual once they have uttered the magic words that they are Not A Doctor. But just because they do not know what to do, this does not stop them from believing that they know what the doctor should do—and how they should interrogate the patient. They are now ready to play 'Does He Take Sugar?'

This was the title of a weekly Radio 4 magazine programme that discussed disability issues. It refers to the phenomenon whereby a disabled person, with a perfectly functioning brain, is sat in a wheelchair when a third party—wanting to find out how they take their tea or coffee—directs this inquiry to the carer stood alongside them. This is obviously demeaning and rude. It implies either that the individual lacks the ability to know what they want or, if they do, that their judgement isn't to be trusted.

I recall taking a telephone call from a senior human resources advisor to a UK FTSE 100 company. It was in relation to a troublesome employee who had been referred to me. The advisor wanted me to be very clear about the questions she was expecting me to address during the consultation. 'I want to know why,' she demanded, 'she doesn't feel able to come to the Anyville site. And why she believes that the area manager's email was inappropriate. And why,' she continued, building to a frenzy of righteous anger, 'she won't talk to me!' After a momentary pause, and the inescapable feeling that I didn't much want to talk to her either, it entered my head to reply, 'I would like to know why you don't feel able to ask her?' There was an awkward pause.

In that instance the manager had only a few questions for me to relay to the individual, but Does He Take Sugar? can often be a lengthy game. The creative manager with time on their hands and an aversion to actually confronting the management issues staring them in the face—matters of attendance, capability and conduct—may devise many tangential questions that they would like their medical advisors to run through with the employee. How long can the employee sit, how many cats do they have, why can't they drive, who mows their lawn, how bad is their headache, why did they make a Facebook posting from a restaurant, how tired do they feel, why hasn't their GP suggested such-and-such a drug, on what dates did they see their GP, why are they going to Dubai for their Christmas holiday, why don't they feel they can work with their colleague, why didn't their specialist arrange an MRI scan, why don't they feel able to undertake telephone duties, who did kill JFK, and so on.

I have seen referrals with over forty questions of this kind, perhaps not asking about the Kennedy assassination but about pretty much everything else. Fifteen to twenty is not uncommon. It is baffling to contemplate how the answers to these questions can possibly help the manager to decide how to manage the employee's incapability, or why—even if the questions are in some way relevant—they feel they need a doctor to ask them on their behalf.

Being the helpful soul that they are, and against their better judgement, the occupational physician will reel off the manager's mindless list of questions and dutifully record the responses given. This is generally all they can do in the short time they have with the employee, excluding the opportunity of using the consultation to make the kind of medical assessment that might actually be useful. Then they will relay back to the employer the 'report'—meant more in a secretarial than a medical sense—from this structured interview, effectively scripted by the manager. At this point the manager will protest, 'But you're only saying what they said!', as though the employee is assumed to be lying or is simply too stupid to know how they feel.

And of course, the subtext to the game is that one or both of these things is true, and the doctor is supposed to be clever enough to realise that. A better doctor would have been able to offer some alternative explanation for the employee's domestic arrangements and social media activities, more in keeping with the manager's prejudice of them as a feckless or malingering individual: someone who in truth has nothing wrong with them and does not need any help in order to keep working. Does He Take Sugar? is a futile attempt to avoid situations that would require management to make the mental effort of having to engage and help the employee, by instead attempting to discredit the inconvenient things they might say. This is done by filtering the employee's perspective through an expert who is somehow a human lie-detector, or at least better able to know how the person is feeling than the person themselves. It is almost exclusively a pointless waste of time.

When someone says they feel unwell and are not able to perform a vital part of their job for whatever reason, or cannot bear their manager, the employer would be better dealing with the inconvenient reality that this is how they feel—and making the difficult decisions that may follow—rather than wasting their energy trying to prove that the person does not know their own mind. The inconvenient reality of both human biology and human relationships is that, from time to time, they go wrong—sometimes transiently, sometimes irrevocably. The employer may be demoralised by the perceived mental effort (and legal risk) of addressing the malfunction, but trying to pretend that it does not exist is scarcely any easier in the long run.

Of all those who have attempted to explain how employers should learn to live with our human nature, given that we will never eliminate it, the American physician Nortin Hadler has made the most helpful contribution. Like many ideas that suddenly afford a new perspective on tired old problems, its appeal lies in its simplicity. In 1997 he suggested that, if we are really to minimise the impact of ill health on the economy, then rather than putting all our effort into the Sisyphean task of eliminating human illness, 'the more reasonable and humane quest might be for workplaces that are comfortable when we are well and accommodating when we are ill.'[1]

This was in the context of back pain but it is relevant across the spectrum of human illnesses. It is a theory that conveys the idea that, if employers want their employees at their stations most of the time, they need to design jobs and workplaces that can accommodate all but the most serious of their intermittent glitches. It acknowledges that—at least until the robot economy becomes a reality—managers are working with mysterious, temperamental and unpredictable human beings. Employers who are serious about addressing the costly problem of sickness must recognise that it is in part a design problem: that historically jobs have been engineered without embedding the flexibility and tolerances needed to accommodate the worker's fluctuating states of health. Second, they must acknowledge that human nature won't change and so, if they want a better fit between the worker and the role, it will be the job that needs tweaking.

Providing comfortable and accommodating workplaces can be costly, depending on the job and the physical environment. Is the pursuit of profit compatible with the provision of humane workplaces? The short answer is yes, since not providing them is even more costly.

Comfort is a relative term. Evidently it is not commercially viable to aspire to palatial standards. Not every organisation has the resources of Wolverhampton City Council which, in 2010, pampered its staff with a 'stress relief day' consisting of 'foot rubs, massages and eyebrow threading', 'in full view of people queuing for housing benefits.'[i] But, by the same token, skimping on expenditure is a false economy too. If Hadler is correct, and it is difficult to mount any serious argument that he is not, then sickness levels will be higher in businesses where work is less comfortable and less accommodating, all other things, such as remuneration, being equal. In such an organisation, no amount of clipboard-wielding safety officers or occupational health practitioners will make much of a difference in herding the workers back to work.

Somewhere on the continuum between Strangeways and Wolverhampton City Council will be a happy medium, and currently most employers don't reach it. If they had a wider understanding of illness, beyond the narrow perspective of health and

---

[i] Members of the public unfortunate enough to have to witness such disturbing scenes as 'Council workers ... laid back in chairs having their feet massaged and their eyebrows waxed ... right next to a queue of people waiting for housing benefits' were incandescent. Sadly for the pampered council staff, 'chiefs were forced to pull the rug on the foot-rubbing sessions following complaints from angry residents.' Most agreed with the *Daily Mail* that it had sent the wrong massage. *Daily Mail* (5 November 2010). 'Sending out the wrong massage: Staff at cash-strapped council given foot rubs as people queue for benefits just feet away'.

safety, and a greater appreciation of human nature and the constant day-to-day variation in how resilient we feel, then the true cost of uncomfortable and inflexible workplaces would in turn be better appreciated. The business case for greater investment in premises, equipment and workplace adjustments would then be that much stronger. This is as true in blue-collar workplaces, where the decision might centre around how far to automate and mechanise roles, as it is in white-collar offices, where it may focus on flexible working arrangements and less dogmatic management about how objectives are reached.

It is relatively early days for this kind of flexibility within employment, however. Take for example a recent initiative from the mandarins of the Scottish and Welsh governments, who have been piloting a 'health and wellbeing hour'. Under this scheme their civil servants are freed from the yoke of public servitude for a paid hour each week of 'pursuits dedicated to maintaining or improving their health'. One civil servant who spent their wellbeing hour 'with colleagues ... walking through a shady wood on the outskirts of Aberystwyth admiring wild flowers in bloom' explained that it had left her 'feeling calm, refreshed and ready to face the afternoon's work.'[2]

As it was, the aspirations for this pilot were not economic but related to wellbeing as an end in itself. But how is the private sector supposed to react to such initiatives if, in truth, they are nothing more than paying people to work less as a means of helping them to feel better? Depicting government initiatives of this nature as 'leading by example' is likely to burst blood vessels in the boardrooms of companies running on such thin margins that experiments of this kind would be pure folly for them, and certainly not good for the wellbeing of the staff who might lose their jobs as a result.

If an economic argument were to be used to justify a pilot of this kind, which would make it widely transferable to the private sector, then this would imply that the proper measure of whether an employee is satisfying their contract should be their overall productivity or quality of work, rather than which and how many hours they have spent chained to their desk. If, this approach suggests, the employee has processed twenty-four widgets rather than the usual twenty, and to the requisite standard, then who cares if they spent an hour walking in the woods? But would the employees involved in such a pilot see it in those terms if the experiment gave unexpected results—if their productivity or performance standard actually fell, would they be prepared to work unpaid after hours, in order to rectify defective widgets or restore a widget shortfall?

For the moment, wellbeing schemes such as the example cited strike me as being at an immature stage in their development. Often it is not clear whether they are being marketed solely on the grounds of making people feel better—which is fine, for those employers with the resources and the desire to procure them—or as a tool for improving productivity, in which case employers at least deserve a plausible business case before dipping their toes in the water. Wellbeing initiatives introduced with the stated objective of improving productivity can, it seems to me, only be effective in workplaces where there is mutual goodwill and a willingness for some trial and error. In work-to-rule environments, where it is a case of heads-you-win and tails-I-lose for the employer, such initiatives seem unlikely to get off the ground in the first place.

Sometimes the barriers to improving wellbeing are not even about cost; the employer may attempt to justify the discomfort of its employees in the name of aesthetics. I was once shown around the newly built, flagship office of a large employer that was intended as a blueprint for similar buildings across the country. My guide mentioned in passing, on three or four occasions, that, despite such a visible investment of money in the interests of employee welfare—and it was many millions of pounds—there was disgruntlement at the reduction in desks compared with the previous building. There were, she explained, only seventy desks for every 100 employees.

As the tour continued, we passed banks of lockers with stacks of cubby trays alongside them. It was obvious that employees would mournfully waste ten minutes at the beginning of the day filling a tray, as a means of transferring their worldly chattels to whichever inch of territory happened to be available, and another ten minutes at the end of the day returning them to their locker. In case this Darwinian struggle for survival were not demoralising enough, it was even marketed to staff using the needlessly emotive term of 'hot-desking'—one that implies the individual would be scalded if they were foolish enough to get at all comfortable and spend too long without moving.

As we walked around, it became clear that this was not a building short on floor space. Bespectacled architects with designer stubble, mood boards and Nordic-sounding names had evidently been hard at work. There were breakout areas, sit-down meeting rooms, stand-up meeting rooms, a wellness room, enormous pot plants, beverage areas, canteen areas and, most of all, space. Acres and acres of painfully chic and opulent open space. It was quickly obvious that there was more than enough floor space for everyone to have a desk. Despite enormous expenditure on a building that the employer calculated staff should want to crawl over broken glass to spend time in, it had managed to disgruntle a sizeable number of them. The morning routine of setting up for work had been transformed into an incessant series of *The Hunger Games*, and all for the sake of the cosmetic appeal of open-plan design.

The inherent wisdom of Hadler's aphorism—that work should be as comfortable as it can be when we are well, and as accommodating as it can be when we are ill—has yet to permeate many workplaces. Rigid patterns of work, inflexible management styles and prescriptive work processes still typify the modern workplace. The norm remains one of straitjacket jobs, only just bearable at the best of times, and periodically intolerable when the humdrum problems of everyday life become just that little bit too much. Many employers recognise that their employees are unhappy and, whilst not quite understanding why, seek to do something to help them. It doesn't occur to them that simply making employees more comfortable by listening to them, believing them, and being pragmatic—loosening the straitjacket—would be a good place to start.

Instead, they think about ways of entertaining the inmates and distracting them from their discomforts. Thus so-called 'wellness interventions' are currently in vogue. They are commoditised solutions such as subsidised gym memberships, tax-free cycle loans, free fruit, and, in businesses that like to think of themselves as funky, full-on kindergarten gimmicks such as ballpools and AstroTurfed offices. Just as the obese have a fondness for diet pills, it is easier for companies to think they can buy a solution to their problems than to consider that they might fundamentally need to change the way they go about things.

Most of the wellness interventions that are dreamt up are unlikely to do much harm. If they make people feel happier, that may be enough for some employers to feel justified in their investment. In well-run organisations they can be the cherry on top, the little flourish of a management team that ultimately knows how to bake a good cake. In organisations that don't 'get' people, however—ones where management is deficient and where the ideas that employees should be respected and work should be comfortable require explanation—then sickness levels will remain high. Fruit smoothies and soft-play are no antidote and will make not a jot of difference.

18

LIMITS TO LAW

Tasks that are ultimately impossible and futile, despite frenetic efforts to achieve them, are sometimes likened to nailing jelly to a wall. However deftly and quickly new nails are hammered in place to restrain the sagging remnants, the gelatinous gloop defies being fixed. Gravity exerts its inexorable pull as lumps work free, stream around their anchors and dribble to the ground. Those who draft statute, and those who establish case law in the courts, are obstinate in their determination to nail down and subjugate the inherent imprecision of language. They are avid and inveterate jelly-nailers.

Just as the quality of sickness defies quantification by doctors, so disability eludes exact definition by lawyers. Both terms are descriptive, qualities that apply to someone to a greater or lesser extent, rather than entities that can be precisely measured. Investigating whether someone is sick or disabled is more like deciding whether they are grumpy or cynical than assessing the evidence of a murder trial, with its dichotomous outcomes of innocence or guilt. It depends: how grumpy or cynical do they need to be before we are satisfied that they reach some arbitrary threshold? How would we ever define in unambiguous terms where that threshold is, and what units should we use to describe it? Is there a particular point on the Meldrew scale of grumpiness to be persuaded that someone is grumpy? How many Udalls does it take to confirm that they are cynical?[i]

Disability does not have a binary, all-or-nothing quality; it is often present to at least some degree on a spectrum that defies adequate human description. At a certain point a notional threshold is reached, where it becomes legitimate to talk about the person as being disabled, but where that point lies is in the eye of the beholder.[ii] Some people, and some tribunal chairs, will require less persuasion than others.

This is a problem for the jelly-nailers. The disability provisions of the Equality Act require employers to exercise positive discrimination—to make 'reasonable adjustments'—for disabled employees. These are intended to help mitigate the effects of the disabling condition that would otherwise prevent the person from being able to work. Examples given in the Code of Practice that accompanies the Act include allocating a disabled parking space, reassigning some aspects of the employee's job for their colleagues to undertake instead, offering flexible working, redeploying the individual to a role they are better suited to, allowing

---

[i] After the notoriously miserable Victor Meldrew, protagonist of the BBC sitcom *One Foot in the Grave*, and the misanthropic Melvin Udall, played by Jack Nicholson in the 1997 film *As Good as It Gets*. Choice lines include Udall's quote to his neighbour, 'You're a disgrace to depression!'

[ii] This is an example of the sorites paradox. If there were a few grains of sand, no one would describe them as a heap. Equally, if there were buckets of the stuff, everyone would agree it was fair to call it a heap. At some point a few grains become a heap, but we cannot define the precise number of grains where this happens and there will never be agreement between different people as to exactly when the transition occurs.

greater time away from work, modifying grievance and disciplinary processes, or adjusting redundancy and performance-related pay arrangements.

These can all be vital in helping severely ill and disabled people to maintain their employment. By the same token, they can all be glittering prizes for the employee to whom it occurs to medicalise their incapability and their dissatisfaction with a manager's unwillingness to overlook it.[iii]

Even the trigger-happy legislators would presumably concede that if employers owe a duty to a specific subset of employees, it is only cricket that they are given some means of confidently deciding which of their employees are disabled. Even more so if the duty is as broad and demanding as having to make all adjustments they reasonably can to their 'provisions, criteria and practices'.[iv] Without such a means of discernment, they are in a double bind.

If they require some degree of persuasion that an employee is likely to be disabled before they will make positive discrimination for them—and, on that basis, do not accommodate everyone seeking workplace adjustment—then there is a good chance that

---

[iii] I work with organisations where this is endemic, and with managers who cannot recall the last time an incapability case did not involve an employee claim of disability and request for reasonable adjustments.

[iv] When considering what adjustments they could make to a role in order to accommodate an employee who may or may not be disabled (much of the time the employer cannot be sure), the law requires that they consider every conceivable aspect of the person's employment where they could potentially intervene. In complex environments and organisations, this can be time-consuming and distracting to say the least. The legislators are ambitious about the extent of the employer's capacity to undertake such investigations, but then most of them have little experience of ever having run a business.

they will periodically be called to the employment tribunal to defend an allegation of failure to make reasonable adjustment. Fairly regularly, they will lose, with all the cost and reputational harm that entails. On the other hand, they may apply a lax approach, where the benefit of the doubt is given to anyone with all but the mildest illness. The danger then is that incapability or poor conduct that is the consequence of incompetence, poor character or lack of work ethic is indulged with excessive sympathy, for fear that in tribunal the poor performance might instead be seen as a feature of a disability, and something that the employer should have adjusted for.

In short, employers need a reliable guide to who is and who is not likely to be disabled—but they do not have one. The statute states that, for a person's condition to be classed as a disability, it must give rise to 'long-term and substantial adverse effect on their ability to carry out normal day-to-day activities.' Long-term is taken to mean that the condition has lasted, or is likely to last, at least twelve months, or for the rest of the person's life if the condition is a terminal one and they are not expected to live that long. Here, at least, we may feel there is some clarity for the employer, 'likely' being a term that most would understand as meaning more probable than not.

But, no. Dictionary definitions of words are often unsatisfactory to lawyers as they make the legal code more directly accessible to the layman. An element of mystery and suspense is introduced by giving them alternative meanings. In this instance, tribunals interpret the word 'likely' as meaning 'might well happen', rather than simply 'more likely than not'. Evidently the range of things that might well happen is far wider than those things that will probably—or, to use the English, are likely to—happen. Most illnesses in most people are short-lived, but there are always exceptions meaning that they 'might well' not be. The majority of people recover from bone fractures, but in a minority of cases persistent malunion can give rise to long-term disability. Few conditions have such a predictable natural history that the doctor is able to offer the patient a reliable guarantee of improvement.

The most slippery word in this definition of disability, though, is 'substantial'. This is self-evidently very subjective and requires amplification. Fortunately, the jelly-nailers have been happy to oblige. Substantial, we are solemnly told, means something that is other than trivial or minor. What is trivial or minor, though, the exasperated employer might well implore—to which the response of their counsel will of course be: something that is not substantial.

There are many other perversities in the legal attempt to define disability. A common mistake among employers trying to use logic and reason to decide if an employee is disabled is to forget that the effects of ongoing treatment need to be discounted when considering the employee's functional ability. If the individual is taking tablets, for example, then it is not good enough to say that they seem okay and therefore are not disabled. The legal definition of disability means that we need to imagine how they would be if they weren't taking the tablets, and whether they would still be okay then.

In a medicalised society, a high proportion of the population are medicated. That proportion will be even higher among the subset of employees seeking adjustment from their employer. So, most of the time, any assessment of the individual by the employer, the occupational health physician or the tribunal is necessarily hypothetical. The person cannot be assessed as they actually are, but as they would be if they had not been given treatment.

In many cases, the medicalisation of the employee is inappropriate and their treatment unnecessary, but that is beside the point. The waters have been muddied, and as a result the individual is that much more likely to be considered disabled.

Take the stressed employee, whose problems exist not in any identifiable medical sense, but in their relationship with their employer—perhaps because they cannot cope with the job that they are engaged to perform, and the employer has taken exception to that. Despite the circumstantial nature of their problems, their despairing GP may well have offered them antidepressant treatment anyway, in an effort to do something tangible in their 600 seconds with the patient. Sometime later, the employee petitions that they have been subject to disability discrimination. Specifically, they allege that the failure of their employer to amend expectations for the role so as to bring it in line with their capability constitutes a failure to make reasonable adjustment. When a tribunal has to assess the merits of the individual's claim, the first consideration will be whether they are actually disabled. Since the effects of ongoing treatment must be discounted, the tribunal's view as to the magnitude of any effect of the GP's nostrum becomes critical. In effect, the tribunal must sit in judgment not just of the employer, but of the prescribing practices of the doctor.

It is one thing to say that someone is not actually disabled, in the sense that there does not seem to be substantial adverse effect on their ability to carry out normal day-to-day activities. But to say that they would still not be disabled even had their doctor not prescribed them antidepressants is to imply poor medical practice. Psychotropic drugs have side-effects and should be dispensed with caution. If their effect is considered to have been so marginal that the person would not be substantially impaired even if they had not been prescribed, then the decision to prescribe begins to look like poor medical practice—which is what it often is.

Proper application of the law then often requires tribunals to adopt a more measured and rational approach to issues of therapeutics than doctors do, and after the event. Tribunals may recognise that they are well out of their depth and in need of medical opinion on the point. But the doctor who issued the offending prescription is unlikely to state that, on reflection, it was probably an instance of malpractice. Should the tribunal ask any other doctor to give a view, that advisor would be hamstrung by the fact that they were not there to make a contemporaneous assessment of the individual—which makes it difficult for them to second-guess with any credibility the treating doctor who was.

Most people recognise the potency of mind-altering drugs, so it is not such an outlandish idea that they might make the difference between someone being disabled or not. What about other interventions, such as talking therapies? In the case of *Kapadia v. London Borough of Lambeth*, the evidence of 'the medical men called on behalf of the appellant' persuaded the Employment Appeal Tribunal that—in a case where the presence of significant adverse impairment was debatable—the fact that the individual had had counselling sessions was sufficient to tip the balance. The Appeal Tribunal concluded that had Mr Kapadia, an accountant for the Borough, not had these sessions, then 'there would have been a very strong likelihood of total mental breakdown and the need for psychiatric treatment including in-patient treatment', and thus that he satisfied the legal test of disability.[1]

Whatever the circumstances in the particular case of Kapadia, the lesson for the disgruntled employee seeking vengeance on their (ex)employer is clear. They would be well advised to exploit the confidential counselling service that most employers provide—and to obtain a script from their GP, which should not be too difficult—before grinding their axe in the Employment Tribunal. It is a brave employer who then contests the issue of their disability. Thus medicalisation can drive legalisation too.

There are other pitfalls for the unwary employer unwise enough to try and robustly establish whether an employee is disabled, rather than simply assuming that they are and adopting the brace position. The statute cites, arbitrarily, conditions that are automatically considered to be disabilities from the point of diagnosis: cancer, multiple sclerosis and HIV infection. It also provides an eclectic list of those that categorically cannot be considered a disability: tendencies to arson, theft, voyeurism, exhibitionism, and the physical or sexual abuse of others. Also, less excitingly, hayfever. Addiction to or dependence on alcohol or other substances is also specifically exempted from the legislation, although its consequences are not. The liver disease and depression of the alcoholic can amount to disabilities, even if the compulsion to imbibe cannot.

Once the statute attempted to define 'normal day-to-day activities', but eventually even the lawmakers recognised that here they had bitten off more than they could linguistically chew. No attempt is made to define what these might be within the current legislation (as of late 2018). The guidance offered by the Office for Disability Issues teaches that watch repair and playing the piano are not day-to-day activities, for those who might have been curious.[2]

Jelly-nailers have a Newtonian clockwork view of the world. They are confident that, with enough careful engineering, things can be made to tick perfectly. They thrive in the bureaucracy of the executive and the legal system, where the delusional belief prevails that subtle concepts can be pinned down through sufficiently careful use of language. Their efforts, as Wittgenstein would have predicted, are self-defeating. Even they, whose very purpose in life is to spend aeons drafting ever more complex iterations of the law, will never succeed in making a definitive description of it. What hope, then, for the citizens—those poor saps required to familiarise themselves with, and apply, the fruits of these legal labours alongside doing their day job?

There is no shortage of helpful guidance for those trying to stay on the right side of the law whilst also trying to run their

236

businesses. The Office for Disability Issues has issued a handy fifty-nine-page guide about 'matters to be taken into account in determining questions relating to the definition of disability' for the bored manager with nothing else to entertain them.[3] That is, if they have any questions left after perusing the Equality and Human Rights Commission's 323-page code of practice in relation to the employment provisions of the Equality Act 2010.[4]

The attempt to define disability in such a way that claims to disability can be consistently tested has been a patent failure. There has been mission creep, because the trend of medicalisation, and the move away from a disease-based conception of illness to one based on how people feel, is just as apparent in the tribunal as in the GP surgery.

When the tribunal receives a claim of disability discrimination, it will, in the first instance, set about deciding if the employee is in fact disabled. In the main this will depend on how the person chooses to report their experience of their symptoms, and they will have had plenty of legal coaching along the way as to the kind of account they might wish to give. If they are on treatment, as most are, then so much the better—since that makes the whole exercise hypothetical anyway. In my estimation, a convincing case for disablement—in the statutory sense—could be made for about 50 per cent of the population, with little ingenuity being required.

Many savvy employers recognised some time ago that, when it comes to disability discrimination, the jig is up. These are typically the larger organisations, or those that have been bruised once too often in tribunal. For them, whether or not an employee is likely to be deemed disabled by a tribunal has become meaningless. The legal definition of disability is simply too unreliable for them to confidently refuse to make adjustments for those employees whom they don't consider to be disabled but who are clearly of a litigious disposition. The employer can only know for sure whether the person actually is disabled when the question is adjudicated in the employment tribunal, by which point it will be too late. If they have contested the disabled status of the individual—and de facto have not made any attempt at positive discrimination—then any claim of failure to make reasonable adjustment will succeed if the tribunal is persuaded that the employee is disabled.

Naturally, some employers have begun to work from the default position that an employee seeking adjustment is disabled until proven otherwise. Aside from my many encounters with large organisations operating on this basis, it is also in keeping with the government's official guidance, specifically paragraph 6.9 of the Employment Statutory Code of Practice accompanying the Equality Act.[5] In these conditions, the management of absenteeism, poor performance or undesirable behaviour becomes fraught. Before the issues can be addressed, managers must consider to what extent 'reasonable adjustments' could be made to every conceivable aspect of the organisation's provisions, criteria and practices. Then, the business case that underpins their decisions must be documented in sufficient detail to satisfy the manager that they could account for themselves if later called to a tribunal. It is an enormous distraction from the job of work, an effective way of engendering compassion fatigue in managers who must demonstrate faux sympathy to all and sundry, and a squandering of the organisation's emotional and financial capital—to the detriment of those who are most seriously ill and in need of the greatest help.

Even then, the curse of the jelly-nailers is not quite dispelled. Just as they cannot make their definition of disability stick to the wall, nor can they cope with the nebulous concept of 'reasonable adjustment'. Again there is guidance—copious guidance—for the insomniac manager, but nothing that is tangible or explicit in helping them to understand quite how far backwards they are required to bend. Section 6.28, on page 85 of the 323-page guide issued by the Equality and Human Rights Commission, explains that reasonableness will depend on various factors. These include the practicability of the adjustment, its likely effectiveness, the associated cost and disruption, the extent of the employer's finances and resources, and the size and nature of the organisation. But, rather like Kentucky Fried Chicken's secret recipe of eleven herbs and spices, the guidance is vague about the suggested quantities of these ingredients. The Commission is as secretive, and as much a tease, as the Colonel himself.

In practice, employers err on the side of caution. Given the disruption brought by tribunal proceedings, the likelihood of losing them on procedural grounds, and the damage to company share prices from a subsequent fall in their environmental, social and governance rating, they know it is best to steer clear of the tribunal. There is little point in making a half-hearted attempt to do so. Sometimes employers go to quite extraordinary lengths in their efforts to avoid a showdown with an employee who has come to be perceived as untouchable.[v] I have known employers to accommodate the sick leave of 'difficult' employees for up to two or three years, rather than argue the seemingly obvious point that no employer can reasonably tolerate someone being away from their work for this length of time.

The disability provisions of the Equality Act are an example of the triumph of intent over consequence. A vague and open-ended duty has been placed on employers towards a very poorly defined group of their employees. This is under threat of fine, public embarrassment and reputational harm to the very same

---

[v] There is a surprisingly widespread belief amongst employees and managers alike that being covered by the disability provisions of the Equality Act renders someone immune to normal management practices, including dismissal.

people whose enterprise and willingness to take risk creates opportunities for employment in the first place. For some in the legislature, the notion that their meddling in the employment relationship can directly threaten jobs and productivity is an abstract one. No doubt there are many disabled people who are now in employment when, without the Act, they would not be. But it is not a safe assumption that the good achieved by its disability provisions has outweighed the harm caused.

Even by its architects' standards, the Act has failed. The rather rosy governmental Impact Assessment of the Equality Act estimated that, after initial setup, the legislation might contribute, in net terms, somewhere between £25 million and £87 million annually to the economy. If this sounds familiar, the reader may be recalling the NHS founders' insistence that it would pay for itself and boost national GDP. But, as with the NHS, it seems that the dream has not come true. Nigel Williams, a statistician for the thinktank Civitas, estimates that, not only was the Act a net debtor to the economy during its first year of implementation, but it is likely to remain so in perpetuity—to the tune of at least £10 million per annum.[6] My own sense, based on my interactions with employers in the years since the Act was introduced in 2010, is that this is a gross underestimate.

I question whether the Act has been particularly effective in achieving equality for disabled people. My experience is that, frequently, the Act's disability provisions have exactly the opposite effect: diverting the effort, money and time of employers towards dealing with those with a profound sense of entitlement—but whose health problems are not notably worse than those of their peers—and away from those with severe and indisputable disability. Since the capacity of any organisation to accommodate disability is finite, any mechanism which purports to target support to a subset of employees most deserving of help, but in practice misallocates this support to a significant proportion who are not, constitutes a disservice to the very group it is intended to help, however noble its stated objective.

Most people would not see cost to the employer as being the principal consideration when the objective is to improve the participation of disabled people in work. Nevertheless it would be Pollyanna-ish to dismiss as wholly irrelevant the drag these disability provisions impose on organisational efficiency, especially if there is also doubt as to their effectiveness. I have seen innumerable cases of management feeling constrained in dealing with intolerable absence, poor capability or behaviours immensely negative to the morale of the wider workforce. This is either for fear of falling foul of the Act, or at least falling foul of the employer's own paranoid interpretation of the duty it confers. This is a paranoia which, in fairness, is not wholly irrational in the context of such bad law and the unexpected outcomes in the lottery of the employment tribunal.[vi] Seemingly straightforward employment relationship problems can prove to be anything but when there is alleged to be an underlying medical problem.

In 2018 there was a Court of Appeal ruling in the case of an English teacher who had been dismissed for having shown a class of 15-year-olds the 18-rated horror film *Halloween*, without consulting the school or parents. The dismissal was deemed to have been unlawful on the grounds that the teacher was debilitated by his cystic fibrosis, and that it was stress—caused by the school's failure to make corresponding reductions in his workload—that had given rise to his error of judgement. The council was ordered to pay £646,000 in damages.[7] Employers reading reports of the case, and seeking to derive learning points from it, will have been struck by how seemingly tenuous the link between the disability

---

[vi] One employment lawyer sets the bar low, when describing the calibre of justice likely to be delivered in tribunal, by cheerfully describing it as the pond life of the justice ecosystem.

and the undesirable behaviour might be. The link between chronic lung disease and a propensity to screen horror movies to teenagers will not be immediately obvious to some of those not present to have heard the evidence first-hand.

These constraints on management decision-making, whether proportionate to the real legal risk or not, generate intangible, pernicious costs which cannot be directly measured. In aggregate across the private and public sector, and up and down the country, I am convinced they amount to a huge sum. Again this perhaps should not be the first concern of disability legislation, but it can scarcely be said to be irrelevant amidst the bemused commentary surrounding Britain's apparently inexplicable productivity problem.[8] In 2017, Chancellor of the Exchequer Philip Hammond had the temerity to make the surely self-evident observation that measures aimed at increasing the participation of disabled workers in the workforce might conceivably also be associated with reduced productivity rates.[9] This was met with a tidal wave of fury and demands that he recant this heresy, with the Green MP Caroline Lucas demanding 'evidence behind his extraordinary claim'.[10] Amidst this outraged grandstanding, one can only assume that the Office for Disability Issues' guide to the definition of disability, or failing that a dictionary, were presumably not to hand.[11]

Nigel Williams of Civitas offers the following thought-provoking summary of the actual consequences of the Equality Act, as distinct from the intended ones:

> By increasing the regulations applicable to businesses, equality legislation risks putting the task of running a business beyond the capabilities of ordinary people. For example, defending or preventing a case against dual discrimination would require knowledge of numeracy, logic and litigation way beyond the essential business skills of producing and selling. Starting a business, one of the traditional paths of social mobility, may be put beyond the reach of people from less affluent backgrounds.[12]

The sick and disabled, and those who think or wish themselves sick and disabled, provide rich pickings for the tribunal-chasers. But we abuse employers at our peril. Whilst there is a widespread stereotype of the employer as a titanic and exploitative bully, whose worst excesses need to be kept in check by the spectre of the tribunals and courts, most employers simply do not have the scale or resources to divert into energy-sapping litigation. They lack in-house counsel and are incentivised to resolve employment disputes as expeditiously and pragmatically as they sensibly can. Our economy is still one dominated by small or medium-sized enterprises (SMEs): businesses employing fewer than 250 staff and with an annual turnover of less than £50 million. Sixty per cent of all people employed within the private sector work within SMEs; they account for 99.9% of private-sector businesses. A remarkable 99.3% of the latter are 'small', companies with no more than fifty staff.[13]

Some years ago, I attended a lecture where I heard a lawyer expound earnestly on the many curious, absurd and contradictory features of disability legislation. Since he invited questions and comments at the end, I suggested that the legal profession had shown a carelessness for the health of the economy that sustained it. My accusations were twofold. First, that the law failed to clarify for employers to whom exactly they owed this additional duty of positive discrimination. Second, that there was enormous ambiguity as to how far this duty might go. As a result, pointless litigation was rife.

A better system could be sketched out on the back of a beer mat. As things stand, attempts to validate and quantify disability are as futile as efforts to measure sickness, and should be dispensed with entirely. As it is, sensible employers are already approaching all cases of ill health on the pragmatic basis that they should do what they reasonably can to help people who are poorly. Whether the employee is in fact considered to be dis-

SICK-NOTE BRITAIN

abled in law—if and when the question is decided in the lottery of an employment tribunal—has become academic. Also, the extent of the duty could be made much clearer with reference to something tangible and objective—namely the average salary within the organisation, a proxy measure for the scale of the employer's resources.[vii]

Defining reasonable adjustments could then be achieved through statute as follows: once the costs associated with an employee's ill health reach, say, 25 per cent of the average salary pro rata, the legal balance would tilt in the employer's favour. In other words, if the sum total cost of the employee's ill health[viii] exceeded a defined percentage of this average salary and the employer subsequently dismissed them, the onus would be on the employee to demonstrate that this was not reasonable, rather than on the employer to prove that it was. Likewise, until the point where costs had reached this level, the employer could expect that a dismissal of the employee would likely be deemed unlawful. Of course, even once an employer had reached the legal limit of their duty, they would retain the discretion to exceed it if they wished—in other words, to work to a best practice approach beyond mere statutory compliance. Incentives encouraging them to do so might be considered, such as reductions in corporation tax rate for businesses recognised as having an exemplary approach to recruitment and retention of disabled staff.

[vii] Disabled employees are already a disadvantaged group within the workplace, hence the desire for disability legislation to redress this imbalance. Using the organisation's average salary—rather than the employee's actual salary—to determine the extent of the duty to make reasonable adjustment would benefit those in lower-paid and part-time roles, who are likely to be the most disabled employees.

[viii] Their sick pay, the costs of covering their absence, and the cost of lost output if they're having to work fewer hours or more slowly than usual.

Clearly this is a proposal that would need refinement—its drafting might require a few more beermats. To what extent should the size of the employer be taken into consideration? There could be a sliding tariff to take into account larger organisations' greater capacity to tolerate sickness. For example, the cost that the employer would be expected to tolerate, as a percentage of their average salary, could be 10 per cent for SMEs with fewer than ten employees, but might be as high as 40 per cent in larger organisations employing more than 1,000. There would also need to be consideration of timescales. How long might the employee need to be in the red, in terms of their net cost to the organisation, before the employer could act with relative impunity if they wished to? The minimum period might also vary with size; perhaps two months for smaller employers but six months for larger ones.

Other quandaries would need to be addressed. In isolation, efforts to regulate just one type of disability discrimination claim—failure to make reasonable adjustment—would fail. If the scope for this particular kind of claim were to be regulated within sensible limits, then the lawyers' ability to exploit other avenues instead—as a means of feeding and educating their children—should not be underestimated. Many cases would simply reach tribunal on other grounds since, as well as providing protection from failure to make reasonable adjustments, the Equality Act provides disabled people with other forms of redress: through the concepts of direct discrimination and 'discrimination arising from disability'.

Direct discrimination is when somebody is treated negatively— for example, is abused, harassed or denied employment—solely and directly on the basis of them having a particular protected characteristic. Direct discrimination occurs not because the employer is concerned (rightly or wrongly) about the consequences of the protected characteristic on the person's ability to perform their role, but purely and simply on the grounds that the person has that characteristic, and the employer's attitude towards such people is negative and prejudicial. As such—if the law deems direct discrimination to have occurred—it is treated as a hate crime, an offence for which there can be no justification.

The Equality Act already incorporates the concept that direct discrimination can be perceptive. It is unlawful for an employer to deny employment to someone because they think that the applicant is gay; whether or not that person actually is gay is beside the point. Similarly, it is an offence for someone to directly discriminate against another person simply because they perceive them to be disabled, irrespective of whether that person in reality satisfies the legal definition of disability. In practice, as we have explored above, the definition of disability is not fit for purpose. Fortunately, even if we were to discard it, the concept of perceptive discrimination means that disabled people would not lose their existing protection from direct discrimination.

Discrimination arising from disability is when the 'provisions, criteria and practices' (PCPs) of an employer have the effect of disadvantaging disabled people, and in a manner that is disproportionate and therefore unlawful. As this definition implies, PCPs can have the effect of disadvantaging disabled people, but in a way that is justifiable in law. These may be instances of discrimination in the semantic sense—the employer has treated one person less favourably than another—but not in the legal sense of constituting an offence. An example of proportionate, and therefore lawful, discrimination is the requirement that airline pilots must be able to see well. This is a recruitment policy that disadvantages blind and partially sighted people, but it is also a proportionate means of achieving a legitimate aim: ensuring the safety of passengers. On the other hand, advertising a job on the basis that a driving licence is essential—which excludes people with conditions that may preclude them from holding a licence, such as epilepsy—may not be proportionate if, in reality, the person doing the role could undertake it just as well using other forms of transport.

Discrimination arising from disability is a very broad concept. Practically every single one of an employer's PCPs could conceivably have the effect of discriminating against disabled people in one way or another, as a couple of notable cases illustrate.

Racist language has a profound effect for those on the receiving end. It might seem reasonable, therefore, for an employer to stipulate that such behaviour is never justifiable; that it is the proverbial red line. Yet the case of *Risby v. London Borough of Waltham Forest* demonstrated otherwise.[14] Mr Risby was a paraplegic employee who became angry and frustrated that he could not attend training being held at a location without wheelchair access. In venting his frustration, he loudly made racially offensive comments, and subsequently his employer dismissed him for gross misconduct. The Employment Appeal Tribunal later deemed the dismissal to constitute discrimination arising from disability. They judged that the misconduct that had caused his dismissal only needed to be tangentially related to his disability for his appeal to succeed. The case of the *Halloween* teacher Mr Grosset is similar.

There is concern in some quarters that claims of discrimination arising from disability may be too easy to make already.[15] Under the Equality Act 2010, the volume of such claims is regulated by applying the disability test to plaintiffs. If they are judged not to be disabled, they fall at the first hurdle and their claim cannot proceed. If this test were to be removed—as I advocate—then there would need to be some other mechanism to deter spurious tribunal adventures by individuals calculatedly seeking to exploit the law for financial gain, often egged on by legal advisors.

The solution would be to focus attention not on the plaintiff's disability, which is subjective and thereby difficult to assess, but instead on the PCP being challenged as discriminatory, which is objective and thereby easier to evaluate. Logically, if an individual raises concern that an employer's PCP is unlawful, then that is an allegation that should be adjudicated on the evidence relating to the PCP: specifically, the extent to which it is indeed a proportionate means of achieving a legitimate aim. But, importantly, not according to whether or not the particular plaintiff is deemed to satisfy the legal test for being a disabled person. Shifting the spotlight away from the individual and onto the PCP would not inevitably open the floodgates for frivolous claims. The deterrent would be the costs imposed on plaintiffs in failed applications, and the penalties awarded against them in frivolous ones. Not, as is currently the case, the misapplication of a wholly unreliable threshold test as a precondition to testing the claim that an aspect of the employer's activities is unlawful.

The threshold at which a PCP was deemed to create a disproportionate disadvantage would need to be set suitably high, for fear of binding employers in impossible red tape and thereby interfering too greatly in their ability to operate. The PCP would need to be egregiously unfair to be considered unlawful. If it were even marginally beneficial to the employer's primary responsibility of running their business safely, fairly and effectively, which is their imperative, then the discrimination claim should not succeed. The law would effectively need to recognise that the primary function of an employer offering employment is as a means of providing goods and services in a commercially sustainable way, and that the aim of achieving social inclusion for disabled people—whilst laudable—is secondary to that.

Whatever the finer points, abandoning attempts to define and measure disability, and instead simply giving employers clear definitions as to the limits of their duties towards disabled people, would be a quantum leap from where we are now. As I outlined my beer mat proposal to the legal speaker, who patiently heard me out, a quizzical grin began to form on his face. These were, he humoured me, interesting proposals. But he had to take exception to the premise of my question. With the demeanour of a Cheshire cat, he clarified that, from the lawyer's perspective, there was no such thing as pointless litigation.

SOLUTIONS

19

THE NECESSARY MYTH

Once, supporting the sick was a matter of individual conscience, judgement and religious teaching. It was an act of human charity between individuals with a relationship to one another. In a more complex society of specialised labour, it became a compulsory and anonymous transaction, mediated by employers and the welfare state. People with jobs were required to obtain a certificate from their doctor before they could be paid statutory sick pay, and in order to satisfy their employer about the authenticity of their absence. Those without work had to jump through the hoops and hurdles of the benefits system to access sickness benefits. In either case, sickness became something that had to be assessed and measured with a veneer of objectivity and plausibility to satisfy all parties about the fairness of the process. It became theatre.

For the individual, certification is necessary as a means of legitimising their inactivity to society—their friends, family, colleagues and managers. It may also be a means of assuaging their own sense of guilt. There will be some who are anxious about burdening their employer or their colleagues, and who are reassured by the sick-note that the situation is beyond their gift to change. No doubt there will also be some who know in their heart of hearts that they are actually capable of work and who are able to kid themselves that, if they have been able to persuade their doctor to write a certificate saying otherwise, they are not doing anything wrong.

Sickness certification of employees is considered important by employers as a means of maintaining workplace attendance. This is the modern incarnation of drapetomania. The individual's urge to flee their miserable job—whether or not they realise this is the real issue in their lives—is conceptualised as a medical problem. The expected treatment is that the doctor will refuse to remove the leg-irons and will instead mandate the employee's return to their slave-owner. But the reality is that they are not a slave; they are a counterparty to the employee contract, free either to attempt renegotiation of their arrangement with their employer, or to stay off work and face the consequences, or to embrace the truth behind their sick leave and resign.

Industrialisation changed the nature of work so that it became monotonous and seemingly pointless. Workers became detached from the earthy realities of tilling the soil and then later harvesting the fruits of their labour, or the artisan satisfaction derived from using their imagination and ingenuity to create and craft new things. Making work fulfilling and even enjoyable in an era of mass production would have required a whole new skill-set on the part of managers and supervisors. It demanded a greater emotional intelligence and understanding of the need to engage the worker if the task at hand was not itself enough to do so.

Very few managed to develop these new skills, and the curse of poor management, the British Disease, is with us to this day. There are plenty of managers who require patient explanation of why making work as comfortable as it can be, and treating people with respect and kindness, is important if they want the best out of them—that is, if the argument that these are good things in and of themselves is insufficient. And there are plenty still who will remain unconvinced even once it's laid out for them.

If the modern manager isn't much cop at giving their staff reasons to want to be in work, they aren't much good at discouraging absenteeism either. The jungle of restrictive employment legislation helps to explain why so many managers seem to have such trouble keeping their teams in work. To some extent the perceived threat of the law is real. Disability discrimination legislation in particular makes such a poor job of defining the extent of the employer's duty—and to whom it is owed—that organisations are fearful of managing poor attendance, performance or conduct with the vigour that they feel is appropriate.

Equally, however, to some extent it is an imagined threat, and the paralysis of the employer's normal management processes is a self-inflicted injury. The Employment Tribunal is not the Supreme Court. Relatively petty employment disputes are bound to arise from time to time wherever human beings are working alongside one another. Whilst they are unpleasant and distracting, they are not the end of the world. Any employer with a large number of employees is going to find themselves in tribunal periodically unless they are prepared to wholly relinquish the management prerogative to manage, which includes making decisions that some people will sometimes find disagreeable. Employers who are terrified of finding themselves in tribunal, let alone losing, may consider that the mere fact of a tribunal automatically implies a failure on the part of their managers. It is not surprising that managers working in a climate of fear and scapegoating are not inclined to do much managing.

The real and imagined risks created by modern employment law have had the effect of greatly restricting the manager's ability to wield a stick over those they want to corral into work. This is especially problematic given that they don't have any carrots to tempt them with either. Their repertoire of tactics that would help encourage their staff to want to be in work—either because they enjoy it, or at least because they recognise that not being there will have undesirable consequences—is dismally narrow. Management by medical coercion is sometimes the only pathetic little implement rattling around in their toolbox. They are looking for the doctor to do their job for them and—in the case of self-entitled and aggressive employees—to become the lightning rod for any bad juju that may follow.

Sickness certification is not just of value to the combatant parties to the employment contract, but to the camp followers as well. Trade union representatives will depict a member's certification as evidence of their ill treatment at the hands of the employer even though most of the grown-ups concerned—including the doctors—would concede, behind closed doors, that certificates are ten-a-penny and not hard to come by. Often the member will have a case, but it is demeaned when these meaningless tokens are the evidence waved around in support of it, rather than anything more substantive. Lawyers too will happily prostitute society's misplaced confidence in the perspicacity of doctors to verify and even explain an individual's symptoms. They pretend that sickness certification constitutes meaningful medical evidence—despite all proof to the contrary—and then use it as a means to pursue compensation claims for alleged disability discrimination and personal injury. Doctors are required to play along, both by law[i] and in order to satisfy their expectant patients.

Then there are the politicians. In a democracy, politics are the art of devising a manifesto that is likely to have the greatest appeal to the greatest number of people, and then persuading

---

[i] Doctors providing primary medical services under the National Health Services Acts are required under the Social Security Acts to issue sick-notes for patients in their care.

them to vote for it. Some votes can be earnt through oratory and persuasion, but fundamentally politicians, like all salespeople, need an appealing product. They pander to the prejudices of their electorate. But sickness throws a spanner in the works for candidates trying to appeal to every man, woman and their dog, because it tends to polarise opinion so powerfully between the hawks and the doves. This is awkward for the aspiring member of Parliament who wants votes from both sets. Each member of the electorate exists somewhere on a spectrum of altruism, from a selflessness to rival Mother Teresa to the self-interest of Gordon Gekko. Those at one extreme expect generous and compassionate sickness policy. At the other end are those who believe that there are no saints, and that all benefit claimants deserve horsewhipping. What is the aspiring politician, trying to gather votes from all and sundry, to do?

The fraud of sickness assessment is the means by which this particular circle is squared. By maintaining the pretence that the saints can be separated from the sinners, politicians can hope to appeal to all quarters of the electorate. The message to the softer souls is: don't worry, we will identify those in need. And, to the diehard cynics: don't worry, we will weed out the scroungers. It is beside the point that this conception of state sickness benefit applicants as either heroes or villains is a nonsense in most cases. This is the way in which much of the electorate views the problem, and to garner support the politician must deal with that perception, rather than the reality.

In the same way, by pretending that there is a reliable means of distinguishing the two groups, politicians also exploit the electorate's prevailing confidence in doctors. They need *The Citadel*'s Dr Mansons, their unimpeachable disability assessors roped in to conduct their wretched Work Capability Assessments, just as Willy Wonka needed the squirrels in his chocolate factory. All are imagined to be frenetically sorting bad nuts from good. Sickness certification of the employed—determining their right to Statutory Sick Pay—serves the same purpose. The softies will be reassured that the underdog worker is protected by being given a piece of paper to wave in the face of their cold-hearted employer. The puritans will be relieved that shirkers seeking more than a week away from work will be put through their paces before it's granted.

Everyone, it seems, has something to gain from sickness certification, except for the besieged doctors in the middle of it all. Clearly this is an inappropriate place for them to be, and we need better solutions to the sickness crisis—but before exploring these, it is worth revisiting briefly the reasons why change is so urgently necessary.

Firstly, the central purpose of doctors is to treat the ill. Because of our society's widespread but irrational faith in their paternalistic wisdom, sickness certification takes them away from this, at a time when pressures on resources are more acute than ever. Sickness absence data since the creation of the NHS in 1948, and studies revealing doctors' approach to certification, provide the evidence that doctors take the path of least resistance. Ethically, it is difficult to expect them to do anything else, given the queues in the waiting room. Confronting requests for inappropriate certification is a time-consuming and largely unsuccessful affair that prevents doctors from caring for those patients who need them most, and they resent being forced between employer and employee to settle what is ultimately a contractual disagreement that both parties are keen to avoid confronting themselves.

Secondly, as necessary as it may be to the agenda of each player in this game, the idea that doctors can reliably disprove an individual's account of being medically incapable is mythical. Medical training imparts skills of disease detection, not illness verification. Many of the ill have nothing objectively 'wrong' with them that can be assessed or measured,[1] by doctors or any-one else. In fact, diagnosis of many illnesses today—and their existence is not in serious dispute—depends on normal test results, excluding the presence of disease. Even when disease is present, this doesn't tell us how the person feels or whether they can do their job. Test results alone are next to useless in predict-ing the extent to which a patient will be disabled by their condi-tion. The cardiologist simply cannot say from a coronary angio-gram how bad their patient's angina is; the orthopaedic surgeon cannot tell the severity of back pain from looking at an MRI scan of the spine. One of the favourite aphorisms of medical educators is that doctors must learn to treat their patients, and not their test results.

What affects an individual's capacity to work is their symp-toms, which they alone can describe and assess in terms of their implications for work. Sickness certification is a shibboleth. Claimants fall into two categories: either they are in the minor-ity group[2] of the very obviously disabled—in which case any-body, medically trained or not, can identify their inability to work; or the case is less clear, and we have only the sick per-son's account of their own experience with which to interpret their capability. In those cases, what is actually in question is an individual's credibility, which doctors are no better placed than others to judge.

Not only that, but they may even be particularly poor candi-dates for the job. They are more likely to be exceptionally altru-istic and trusting of their patients—as they are trained to be—than exceptionally cynical or combative, as fraud investigators must be. Every medical student is at some point taught the apho-rism that '80 per cent of diagnosis is in the history', meaning that in clinical practice they will make 80 per cent of their diag-noses on the basis of what their patients tell them—rather than according to anything they can find on physical examination or in test results.[ii]/3 Doctors are conditioned to attach great value to what the patient relays to them; taught that, within the oddities, incongruities and throwaway remarks of the story they are given, there may well be the clue to an otherwise elusive diagnosis. They are loath to disregard what their patients have to say to them, still less to suspect that patients are intentionally leading them astray.

Also, the architects of the sickness certification system are lawyers and politicians (a disproportionate number of the latter having previously been lawyers). Challenging the integrity of witnesses is second nature to lawyers: it is the bread and butter of litigation. They mistakenly assume that doctors operate with similar latitude. But the legalisation of our society means that questioning a patient's integrity will only invite the medical regulator into the fray. That should be no surprise, because disbelief and accusations simply do not constitute the kind of dynamic that society considers acceptable between sick people and their healers. Their job is poles apart from that of the sickness certification brief.

Finally, even if, against all odds, doctors were to embrace the interrogative nature of certification, they could not do so effectively, because they can only assess claimants aware that they are being observed. There are extraordinary examples of doctors whose sense of public conscience has overcome their sense of professional self-preservation, but they are few, and unlike Dr Manson they are not lauded for it. In 2006, the West Midlands Police psychiatrist Dr Nicholas Cooling was suspended

---

[ii] The aphorism seems to have its origins in a *BMJ* paper from 1975 by Hampton et al., where a series of 80 patients who had been referred to medical outpatients by their GPs were followed up. In 66 of the 80 cases (83%), the diagnosis initially made on the basis of the patient's history was unchanged even when further information—examination findings and test results—became available.

for two months by the General Medical Council after arranging for a private detective agency to undertake surveillance of an officer whom he suspected of malingering. At his GMC hearing, Cooling was admonished for misconduct amounting 'to a breach of one of the fundamental tenets for medical practitioners.'4 When benefit fraudsters are convicted in the courts, it is invariably on the basis of video footage. But we don't judge it acceptable for doctors to obtain such evidence; covert surveillance is the remit of the forensic investigator, while value-judgements about a person's credibility are the responsibility of the judiciary.

The attempt to shoe-horn doctors into a role that doesn't fit them has caused much harm. This has been to individuals, who are infantilised; to our politics, which are subverted; to our economy, as much avoidable sickness is caused by doctors; and to our health service, because, as its embattled state illustrates, there are more useful things doctors could be doing. Embroiling them in the politics of sickness has proved to be a costly accident of history.

All this is not to say that doctors have no role at all in reducing the level of sickness within society. Removal of the certification function would not change the fact that doctors are the key source of health advice for the patients who consult them. If it were the case that work was generally detrimental to health and wellbeing, then there would be a problem, as the primary ethical duty of the doctor is to the person sat in front of them. The advice they would need to give in those circumstances would not be conducive to maximising national GDP. Fortunately, the great majority of the time—except in rare cases where there is serious medical risk, or the patient is so ill that they could not manage even heavily modified work—there is extensive evidence that being in work is generally good for people. The activity, routine, distraction, socialisation and opportunities for career progression and social mobility all tend to help people who are well to stay well, and people who are ill to get better. Medical advice to the individual that they should remain in work as best they can, and return as soon as possible if they have fallen out of it, is good advice for the patient as much as it is helpful to the interests of the wider economy.

When doctors are positioned in a way that plays to their strengths—as health educators, trusted advisors and advocates—they can achieve a great deal for employees and their employers. Doctors can be persuasive and effective in changing the thinking and behaviour of the individual, in challenging the mythical ideas that still permeate society about the virtues of rest and the perils of work. Here the inherent altruism common to many doctors, and the emotional intelligence and communication skills honed by their training and daily work, is of valuable use. Society still places great trust in doctors, which further enhances their ability to assert leverage over those who consult them.

To be most effective in this advocacy role, patients must believe that the doctor is acting with integrity and solely with their interests in mind. One of the ironies of certification is that it undermines the trust that patients would normally have in the advice of their doctor by introducing a conflict of interest. It seeds a nagging doubt in the patient's mind as to whether what is being said is really being said because it is true, or because it is what the doctor's paymasters expect them to say. The certification process per se actively undermines doctors in their ability to do what they are good at, whilst requiring them to do things that they are not good at.

The doctor is not a party to the employment contract. It is not for them to dictate to the employee how much suffering they should endure before they decide that not attending work is preferable to soldiering on, if the consequences of that choice are loss of pay and potentially loss of job. How the pros and cons weigh up is a matter for the individual, and they should be afforded the dignity of exercising their own choice. Nor is it for the doctor to decide on behalf of the employer what minimum level of work they should expect for the employee's pay and rations. That is something the employer must make their own decision about, according to the commercial circumstances and the extent of their corporate benevolence. When the plain truth is that the employer has decided that enough is enough, and that an ill employee needs to be dismissed, they should no more hide behind the writ of the doctor—seeking their declaration that the worker is 'unfit'—than an absent employee should maintain that it is their doctor's doing that they are not attending work.

Fundamentally, doctors do not write the rules of the employment contract; nor do they enforce them. It is a mistake for either of its actual parties to look to the doctor to arbitrate the breach of contract that arises when, for reasons of illness, the employee is not able to uphold their part of the bargain. Doctors have about as much business advising employers what to do in these situations as they would have advising employees about what they should do in the event that the employer's payroll system were to crash. In either case, the issue is one of contractual frustration. These situations are important to the signatories to the employment contract, but they are not a direct concern of the doctor.

That said, when ill health means that the employee is struggling to cope—and when the employer has been clear about how far the bar can be lowered for them—doctors are amongst the best people who can enthuse and train the individual so that they have the best chance of coming up to scratch. Doctors come into their own when they are not being asked to draft or enforce the rules of the employment game, but to help the players to do what the team manager requires. They make terrible referees, but excellent coaches.

20

THE LEAP OF FAITH

The entire history of medicine has been characterised by the desire of individuals to seek easy, purchasable answers to life's woes, and of medicine's wiser practitioners—who recognise that these treatments are frequently counterproductive—to discourage them from doing so, often not very successfully. Hippocrates said that 'whenever a doctor cannot do good, he must be kept from doing harm', whilst his modern contemporary Sir William Osler observed that 'the first duty of the physician is to educate the masses not to take medicine.' The same is true when it comes to sickness, a complex social ill to which the beguilingly simple solution is sickness certification. In practice, though, certification causes more harm than good and, as with any sham treatment, we would be better off for being weaned from it.

Some fear that if we dispense with the practice of sick certification, hordes of people will stop going to work and the country will grind to a halt. They believe that it is the role of doctors in the primary care system to hold the line, to steadfastly refuse the skivers from gaining access to the ranks of the sick. It is as though every surgery should be a re-enactment of a military skirmish, with the doctors defending the beachhead. Yet the reality—the evidence of history since Lloyd George's first National Insurance Act back in 1911—is that sick certification is largely ineffective in preventing avoidable sickness. Doctors cannot vouch for how someone is feeling any better than anyone else can. Even when they are sceptical, their uniquely difficult ethical, professional and regulatory situation means that they are compelled to hold their tongue. Worse, certification even causes some degree of avoidable sickness.

It leaves people feeling vindicated in their decision not to attend work when, with a little effort by two parties, they probably could. It stops employees and their managers from speaking directly to one another about the problems the individual is experiencing, and the things that could be done to try and help them remain in work. It tends to result in certification for arbitrary periods of time such as a week, a fortnight or month, when, on probabilistic grounds alone, most people's recovery will fall on the days in between and, were it not for an open sick-note, they would otherwise return to work at that point. Abandoning certification would be good news for everyone except the producers of daytime television programmes.

Even if sickness certification is a deterrent to avoidable sickness to any extent, this is simply not the role of a primary care system—especially one that already cannot meet the demand for its core function, which is the assessment and treatment of illness. It cannot be right that, at a time when patients are having to wait, on average, approximately a fortnight to see their doctor, anywhere between a tenth to a third of consultations are being used to issue sick-notes (see Chapter 9). It is not the responsibility of doctors to enforce the attendance of employees in jobs that, because of lack of care and effective leadership from their employer, they don't enjoy or find unreasonably difficult. Nor to help the employer circumvent their fears of managing absence or incapability, stoked by the efforts of lawyers in creating a legal landscape that managers perceive as hopelessly complex and impossible to navigate. These are contractual and legal concerns, not medical ones.

Others reason that certification has an important role in protecting vulnerable people from exploitation. Some may fear that, without the scrap of paper from their doctor, these employees may be compelled to attend work in circumstances where it is just unreasonable to expect them to do so. But the removal of certification is not the removal of access to advice from a trusted GP. Doctors would remain quite able to advise patients about their choices regarding work, as they always have. Where the employer's actions might be construed as bullying, this support from the GP might include signposting to organisations such as Citizens Advice for legal advice. Mandating certification for the entire working-age population on the grounds that there are some bullying and unscrupulous employers is applying a medical sledgehammer to crack a legal nut.

Then there is the concern that removing certification would expose workers to risks of harm from their employment. Fears about the hazards of work are commonplace, part of our cultural DNA, but they are out of all proportion to reality now that most people work in service roles in our post-industrial economy, under all the protection offered by health and safety legislation. The current certification process undoubtedly exposes more people to risk than it protects from injury, by increasing the chance that they will fall out of work, with all the health risks this entails. Where employees are concerned that their job poses a risk to their health, again, abolishing certification would not prevent them from seeking their doctor's advice about the extent of this risk.

In safety-critical roles—where there would be a risk of substantial harm to the individual, or to others, if they were working whilst unwell—the current certification system is in any case an insufficient safeguard. It relies on the individual recognising that there may be a problem, then consulting their doctor, telling them the truth, accurately reporting the nature of their job, and relaying the opinion of the doctor—the sick-note—back to their employer. As a safety-management system it has more holes than a Swiss cheese. To avoid depending on the employee to flag a health issue, additional safeguards are used, with occupational physicians—knowledgeable about the role, its risks, and the ways in which health problems might interact with these—periodically assessing employees. However, even these systems still rely on effective and honest communication between multiple parties, and incidents such as the Glasgow bin lorry crash in late 2014 or the Germanwings disaster in the spring of 2015 are examples of the tragedies that can occur when this communication fails.[1]

The fitness assessment system for high-risk industries could be further strengthened by ensuring that, when an individual is appointed to such a role, the new employer notifies the employee's GP. The employer would provide them with details of the organisation's occupational physician, whom the GP should contact in order to discuss in medical confidence any concerns that later arise about the patient's fitness. The definitive decision about fitness would then be a matter for the occupational physician, who is suitably trained, knowledgeable and experienced to make an appropriate assessment of the medical risk. And, as always, the employee should only carry out their safety-critical duties if they consider that they are fit and safe to do so, irrespective of the drawbacks for them if they do not. This enhanced safety system can be described as a triple-lock, as the individual is only engaged in safety-critical activity if all three parties—they themselves, their GP, and their occupational physician—are simultaneously in agreement that they are fit to do so.

Arguably medical processes specifically intended to reduce the risk of harm from ill health in the workplace can have the opposite effect. The external affirmation of an employee's (un)fitness to work—whether in the form of a certificate of fitness, or a sick-note—may leave the line manager feeling overly reassured, or unwilling to raise their own concerns about the employee's safety. This could be out of intellectual laziness, cowardice, or an error of logic telling them that their view is immaterial, due to their lack of medical training. I recall receiving a referral for an employee driving heavy plant who had already been involved in a series of accidents, and whose manager described him as 'one job away from a serious accident'. I was astonished to learn that management were still allowing him to drive pending his medical assessment, as they felt that they could not justify standing him down without an assessment outcome in that direction. Such instances, while perhaps not common, are not exactly rare, either. More recently, I saw a referral where the same dynamic was at play, this time relating to an offshore worker—an especially hazardous environment—about whom a number of colleagues had already raised safety concerns.

To give an example where the risk of harm was realised, in October 2015 a double-deck bus was driven by its seventy-seven-year-old driver off the road and into a Sainsbury's store, killing a seven-year-old boy sat at the front of the upper deck and a seventy-six-year-old pedestrian. It later emerged that, prior to the crash, the bus company had sent this driver no fewer than eight warning letters, triggered by the accelerometer's detection of erratic driving. The warning letters had resulted in him being referred to the company's driving school for a reassessment, which concluded that his driving was 'uncomfortable and erratic' and 'would not have been good enough' to pass an initial driving test. By the time of the trial, he had been diagnosed with dementia and was unfit to plead.[2] As a driver aged over seventy, this man will have been assessed yearly in a D4 medical, as required by the DVLA. We can speculate that the fact of these annual medicals might have provided a false sense of reassurance as to the driver's fitness to continue working in between them, despite the manifestation of symptoms.

Satisfaction of medical fitness standards is necessary but not, in and of itself, sufficient evidence of safe capability in a safety-critical role. I might pass a pilot's medical, but you assuredly would not want to get on a plane controlled by me. In effect, therefore, the most appropriate solution is a 'quadruple lock': not only the employee and the doctors involved, but also the manager—whose job it is to have a view on the individual's capability in their role—must also be content that the employee remains fit to work. If we were to dispense with the current system of sickness certification, and replace it with the enhanced system I have described, a crucial part of its safe implementation would be to ensure education of managers to understand that their assessment remains critically important, even when both doctors agree that the individual is fit. In a safety-oriented system—because we are only talking about certification of high-risk roles—the concerns of any one of the four would veto the reassurances of the other three, and remove the employee from work until the matter was resolved. One might think that such logic should be self-apparent, but concerning examples such as the above illustrate that this is not always the case.

Quite apart from the practical, logistical, financial and safety arguments for abandoning the century-old practice of sickness certification only by GPs, there is an ethical one. We live in a time when we have rejected medical paternalism, and invoke the right of the individual to make decisions about all aspects of their life including their medical care and treatment. It is bizarre that we still require the writ of the doctor to mandate a decision as important as whether or not we feel fit to go to work in an era when, if a doctor were to insist that a patient took a particular treatment, we would view it as an unforgivable infringement of the individual's autonomy. It is a regressive and infantilising throwback to a time when the power balance in the relationship between worker and employer, and patient and doctor, was very different. We would all be better off for growing out of it.

There are some policy changes that could be made in conjunction with any plan to abolish the certification system, to ease our transition from kindergarten into this grown-up world. The greater requirement for managers to deal directly with absent employees would mean that the need for better manager training would become acute. This would be not just in terms of the soft skills needed to help support sick employees back into work, but also the tenacity needed to consistently apply the organisation's absence procedures to those truculent absentees demonstrating little appetite for being back at their job.

Since existing employment legislation makes absence management a terrifying prospect for the nervous line manager the legislature could oblige a little here, by loosening some of the employment protections for employees. Especially those relating to disability discrimination, by clarifying the extent of the employer's duty towards disabled employees in the way described earlier in this book. The abandonment of sickness certification would mean that the burden of dealing with absence shifts from the general practitioner to the line manager. It would then be the manager having their feet held reluctantly to the fire; the lawyers could help by at least turning down the heat a little.

Another measure worthy of consideration would be to review arrangements for statutory sick pay, with a view to introducing greater mutuality of interest. The law requires that employers pay a statutory minimum (£92.05 per week as of 2018) to employees who have been sick for at least 4 days in a row. The employer is entitled to ask for a sick-note beyond the seventh day of absence in order to continue payments, just as a schoolteacher might expect the child suspected of truanting for a note from their parent. Until April 2014 employers could reclaim these payments from HMRC, but that is no longer the case.

The detriment to the absent employee is that they lose pay during the first few 'waiting days', although even this may not be true if it is a recurring absence,[i] and, whilst being paid SSP—to which they are entitled for twenty-eight weeks—their income is likely to be significantly lower than normal. The Office for National Statistics provides data about median weekly earnings across the different occupation types and even the lowest paid group, 'Caring, leisure and other service occupations', receives a median weekly wage of £374.[3] There can be little doubt that, for low-paid workers, falling onto SSP for any length of time can cause real hardship quickly. Even so, employers feel aggrieved that the cost of paying for days when the employee has done no work falls solely on the organisation. This is especially so, of course, in circumstances where they judge that the employee's absence is not genuine. There is something to be said for using National Insurance payments as a means of building an SSP 'pot', in a similar way to how National Insurance payments are used to build the individual's state pension pot.

Employees who rarely took recourse to sick leave would, on reaching state retirement age, be paid a modest nest-egg as some kind of recompense. This would perhaps be fairly token given the sums involved, but symbolic nevertheless. Those who had dipped into the pot more regularly during their working career would receive a smaller sum, and those who had exhausted it entirely would receive nothing at all—though the minimum SSP entitlement during their working life would have to be main-

---

[i] As with all such schemes, things are never quite so simple. SSP may be payable without the employee having to wait a few days first, if they were also off sick—and paid SSP—in a separate period during the preceding 8 weeks.

tained through state top-ups. In this way, conversations about return to work could take place in more of a spirit of mutual co-operation, with both manager and employee being more appreciative of the costs of absence when the burden is more fairly shared. In situations where the employee could feasibly manage some suitably modified work, this system would be a further incentive to them seeking that before going sick. In situations where they could not, it might go some way in improving the empathy of the line manager, since it would be apparent that the employee was having to bear at least some of the cost.

Suggestions about loosening the employment protections for employees who cannot sustain their work, or trying to introduce some greater intelligence into sick pay arrangements, are all very well in theory. In practice, there have been few efforts at sick-note reform since 1911, and these have been rather desultory. In 2010 there was an attempt at rebranding the paperwork, the med3 thereafter referred to as the fit-note rather than the sick-note. This was with the honourable intention of trying to draw everyone's attention to what the person remained able to do, rather than what they couldn't. However, since the statutory purpose of the note remained to authorise the individual's entitlement to SSP, the change in terminology always appeared an Orwellian abuse of the English language, and has not been especially successful.

The newly designed med3 included an option for the doctor to declare that the patient 'may be fit for work taking account of the following advice', followed by some tick-box suggestions for 'a phased return to work', 'amended duties', 'altered hours' and 'workplace adaptations'. This section of the form included space where the certifying doctor could append more specific comments about the kind of adjustments that might be suitable for the convalescent. The intention was that if this led to some fruitful dialogue between the employee and their manager, such that they could identify modified work for the individual, then it might avoid the need for absence altogether. In other words, the hope was that the med3 might be used as an advisory note on some occasions, rather than as evidence of entitlement for SSP.

These hopes have not been fulfilled. One study of 58,695 fit-notes found that the 'may be fit for work' option had been used in just 6 per cent of cases. In a small percentage of these— 7 per cent—though the GP had suggested the individual may be fit for work, they had provided no suggestions as to the kind of adjustment that might be helpful.[4] The problem of course was that merely reformatting the fit-note did nothing to address the most serious problems with the process. Namely, that doctors did not feel trained, competent or confident to undertake certification, nor did they feel it was even an appropriate thing for them to be asked to do—regardless of what paperwork they might be using.

A survey of 1,665 general practitioners, two years after the introduction of the new fit-note, found that they were fairly ambivalent as to its impact.[5] Those who completely disagreed that it had 'increased the frequency with which I recommend a return to work as an aid to patient recovery'—11.1% of the sample—slightly outweighed the 9.7% who completely agreed with that statement. As for those who were fairly nonplussed either way, 50.8% 'somewhat agreed' with the statement, whereas 28.5% 'somewhat disagreed'. Overall, then, the net sentiment of these GPs was that the reforms might have made them marginally more likely to recommend return to work—faint praise indeed.

The May government, disappointed at the limited impact of the 2010 reforms, published a green paper in October 2016 with proposals for further changes to the certification system, which were out for consultation. The green paper included the euphemistic observation—stated more directly half a century ago by

Dr Handfield-Jones—that doctors 'may, on occasion, find it difficult to refuse to issue a fit note'. Though the consultation dared to ask, 'Are doctors best placed to provide work and health information, make a judgement on fitness for work and provide sickness certification?', no suggestion was raised that medicine in general might be ill placed for the task. The follow-up consultation question was: 'If not, which other healthcare professionals do you think should play a role in this process...?' The green paper's overall conclusion was to review 'whether fit note certification should be extended from doctors in primary care and other settings to other healthcare professionals.'[6] Dr Manson may have been hasty in confiscating the pharmacist's stamp.

Naturally enough, the only sensible contribution to the UK debate about certification in recent times has come from its most prominent victims: the general practitioners. In 2005 a survey found that almost half of them believed it inappropriate that GPs were required to issue sick-notes.[7] Unsurprisingly, at the British Medical Association's 2016 Annual Representatives Meeting, a motion that the period of self-certification[ii] should increase from seven to fourteen days was overwhelmingly passed.[8] The deputy chairman of the BMA's GP committee, a Leeds GP, emphasised that the key issues related to trust, and the need to prioritise the therapeutic work of doctors: 'Essentially it's about empowering patients and trusting patients and reducing unnecessary appointments with GPs'. He went on to make the equally reasonable observation that 'If anybody is abusing the system that becomes an issue for their employer.'[9]

The impertinent BMA doctors getting such silly ideas above their station were quickly slapped back down. A representative from Patient Concern likened the proposal to 'a skiver's charter',

---

[ii] The period for which employees are able to claim SSP before needing to obtain a med3.

whilst a DWP spokesman rejected it on the counterfactual grounds that the existing certification system did not overburden general practitioners. The commercial director of a company that sells absence management software—and who was therefore seemingly considered an expert on the work of GPs—provided a straw man by saying that doctors 'want[ed] to reduce their workload', and patronised them with the passive-aggressive recognition that 'they are not the only professionals working in challenging conditions'.[10] This was to misrepresent the issue, since the proposal was not the result of GPs seeking to reduce their workload but to reprioritise it. The demands of dealing with ill people are high enough that GPs would still be in the surgery rather than on the golf course if they were relieved of the obligation to issue notes. Whatever professionals this commentator was comparing them with were presumably being challenged by their own job, and not by inappropriate demands to do someone else's.

If they were hoping for solidarity from other medical quarters, the GPs were to be disappointed. A survey of 122 occupational health professionals found that only 7 per cent agreed with the BMA's proposal to extend self-certification, and only 2 per cent thought it should be extended further.[11] The Faculty of Occupational Medicine, the professional body for occupational physicians, and the Society of Occupational Medicine, an association of all kinds of occupational health professionals—primarily doctors and nurses—issued a joint statement criticising the suggestion.[12] They declared that, whilst they appreciated the strain on family doctors, they believed early conversations between the employee and the GP were important. Yet the fact is that it might be conversations between the employee and their manager, not their doctor, that actually matter most, and that being made to obtain a certificate tends not to facilitate that process but to interfere with it.

Amongst the business community, the Federation of Small Businesses expressed fears that absence levels would soar as drapetomanic employees were allowed to flee their hateful jobs, while the Confederation of British Industry suggested the current system was needed 'to enable employers to understand' the present and future capacity of their sick employee.[13] It is heartening indeed to see such confidence in the UK workforce amongst our business leaders, and in the competence of the management cadre to manage it.

Elsewhere in the world, doctors have made similar pleas for a rational re-evaluation of certification, again to no avail. As we saw in Chapter 9, in 2011 Professor Max Kamien of the University of Western Australia argued that asking doctors to sign sick-notes was a costly waste of time, and best abandoned. His credentials for contributing to the debate are significantly more impressive than those of the naysayers. At the time he made these remarks, he had been a practising doctor for fifty-one years and estimated that he had provided more than 20,000 certificates in that time. The predicament of the Australian doctors is even more acute than that of their British colleagues. In Australia employers can legitimately require a certificate from employees who have had more than two days off sick in any given year.[14] That this remains the case shows that Professor Kamien's intervention fell on deaf ears, just as the BMA's did. It may also help to explain the emergence in 2015 of an online service that Australian employees could use to obtain sick-notes more conveniently, branded with typical Antipodean bluntness and irreverence as Dr Sicknote—later rebranded as the only slightly more palatable Qoctor.[15]

All attempts at tinkering with the certification process, short of making the leap of faith and abandoning such folly entirely, are doomed to failure. This has been the case since Sir Claud Schuster's 1914 inquiry into why the 1911 National Insurance Act had so rapidly and unexpectedly headed off the fiscal rails. It is because the assumptions underpinning such schemes—that sickness can objectively be measured, and that sappy healthcare professionals will somehow prove immune to the conflicts of interest involved—are fatally flawed. No attempts at botching a repair can be effective. This is true whether the proposed reform is to tweak the period of time for which the individual can self-certify, the wording on the paperwork used, or the type of healthcare professional allowed admittance into the nut-sorting room: previously the hallowed ground of doctors alone but, to go by the 2016 green paper and a late 2017 white paper,[16] not for much longer. Soon healthcare professionals of all ranks may get to waste their time too, engaged in the dismal business of certification. The attempts to make sickness certification function effectively over the last century have been like the charge of the Light Brigade: full of sound and fury, but a battle of senseless loss for little gain. The only rational tactical response should be to withdraw. Instead we are preparing to throw more ancillary divisions into the fray.

Attempts at validating sickness are as pointless amongst the unemployed being assessed for state sickness benefits as they are amongst the employed troubling their doctor for a note. All the same arguments apply, merely in a different context—as does the same solution, which is abolition of such assessments, rather than endless tinkering with gaffer tape solutions such as Regulation 35(2)(b). This was the conclusion of the last independent reviewer with the unhappy task of assessing the effectiveness of the Work Capability Assessment for a parliamentary report, who ended by questioning the rationale for the assessments in the first place.

Fortunately, consigning sickness benefit assessments to the dustbin of history does not pose insurmountable problems in terms of how benefits should be administered, because state sickness benefits per se are an anachronism and should go the same way. It is important to question the raison d'être for benefits that are targeted according to an individual's notional health-related capacity for work.

The emergence of state sickness benefits was surprisingly recent. From the Elizabethan Poor Laws of 400 years ago, the Local Government Act of 1929, which transferred the powers of the Poor Law Unions to local authorities, and the National Assistance Act of 1948—in fact, right up until 1971—the relief administered to those not working for reasons of ill health was not distinguished from that given to people not working for any other reason.[17] In other words, in terms of the support provided by the state, whether someone was sick or simply unemployed was largely immaterial: the means-tested assistance they received would be the same in either case.[iii] It was Edward Heath's Conservative government that ushered in the era of state sickness benefits with the introduction of Invalidity Benefit in 1971. This was materially worth more than the standard Unemployment Benefit, and it was this differential—which became more marked over the next couple of decades—that proved so expedient for successive governments keen to keep the unemployment count depressed to an artificially low level.

Around the same time, disability benefits were introduced— 'extra-cost' benefits intended to cover the additional costs that someone living with a disability might face. These were the Attendance Allowance of 1971, for people requiring substantial assistance in their day-to-day lives, and the Mobility Allowance of 1975, for those needing help to get around. Over the next couple of decades, there was a recognition that these benefits were too small to meet the needs of many disabled people, and so in 1992 the more generous Disability Living Allowance was introduced, followed by the Personal Independence Payment of 2013.

[iii] From 1966, though, Supplementary Benefit incorporated a more generous rate of benefit for those out of work long-term, which would have included sick and disabled people.

Against this backdrop, the concept of sickness benefits begins to look shaky. Fundamentally, what does society intend? Is it to provide support for the costly adaptations that a disabled person may need in order to participate in social and working life to the fullest possible extent? The answer must surely be 'yes', and there will always be a consensus for a system of generous benefits to that end: practical and financial support and assistance to overcome the person's functional impairment, irrespective of whether or not they happen to be working. These are disability benefits, not sickness benefits. They are targeted according to the degree of disability, not whether the person is in work. Is the intention of welfare also to prevent abject destitution, however caused, and even if it is in part the fault of the individual? Again, most would say 'yes'—in which case the concept of a universal out-of-work benefit covers all bases. Whether the person is unemployed, sick, feckless or living on the moon is beside the point.

In such a system of coherent and comprehensive benefits, what rationale remains for sickness benefits—benefits solely dependent on assessment of health-related fitness for work? For a claimant who is disabled and happens to be out of work, in receipt of disability and out-of-work benefits respectively, what is the logic for an additional system of sickness benefits? The only argument could be: to compensate for the misfortune of being sick, since the costs of being disabled and the costs of being unemployed would each be satisfied already. Is this wise, and is it what society wants? The answer surely is 'no' on both counts. The perils of incentivising worklessness are obvious to most, even if they are too obvious for some academics. Furthermore, we don't see social insurance as a means of compensating people for bad luck, but rather for the consequences of bad luck, which is subtly different.

The whole concept of sickness benefit can be seen as a wrong turn, an accident of history. The welfare state did not emerge fully formed overnight; it developed piecemeal, like most attempts at progressive reform in developing countries. It is understandable, perhaps inevitable, that sickness would have been identified as a social scourge in its own right sooner or later in the evolution of the welfare state. And, cynically, that sickness benefits would have attracted the attention of cynical politicians keen to disincentivise the uptake of unemployment benefits. But these circumstances are no longer true. For one thing, unemployment levels are historically low, and government has no need to try and disincentivise people without jobs from claiming unemployment benefit. And, as the welfare state has matured, and unemployment and disability benefits have improved, so the need to use sickness as a characteristic for targeting benefit has made progressively less sense. The crude, early attempts at providing sickness benefits forty years ago can be thought of as a redundant scaffold, now that a more substantial infrastructure for social security is in place—in particular, a better system of disability benefits. Today, dismantling the scaffold is the obvious course of action. The appeal of this solution is that it renders wholly academic the impossibility of designing a sickness assessment process that is fit for purpose yet also avoids collateral damage to those we most want to protect from harm.

It is difficult to see who would lose if sickness benefits were to be scrapped, and if the money saved were to be redistributed to sick people through an enhanced system of disability benefits instead, paid in conjunction with existing unemployment benefit. The only losers, perhaps, are the multinational corporates who currently undertake Work Capability Assessments on behalf of the DWP, to the tune of more than £180 million per annum.[18]

Add to that sum the half a billion spent on administering this expenditure[iv]—including £22 million in 2016 on its internal

---

iv The DWP's 2015–16 'Annual Report and Accounts', referenced else-

process for appeals against sanctions, £17 million for contesting cases that have reached tribunal,[19] and the £66 million cost to the Courts and Tribunals Service of hearing ESA appeals,[20] and that is a lot of money: perhaps three-quarters of a billion pounds not reaching sick and disabled people every year. Yet, incredibly, a 2018 Commons Select Committee report into sickness and disability assessments closed with the suggestion not that we should revisit the very principle of these costly and distressing assessments, but instead that the DWP 'may well conclude [that] assessments are better delivered in house'—a quintessential case of missing the wood for the trees.[21]

---

where, revealed that the DWP had operating costs of £6.5bn that year, and distributed £173bn of welfare spending. Spending on ESA (the vast majority of sickness benefits) was £14.5bn. Multiplying ESA expenditure as a percentage of total expenditure by DWP operating costs produces the hypothetical figure of £545m (14.5/173 x 6.5 = 0.545).

21

A SORT OF LIFE

During the nineteenth and twentieth centuries, the battle against occupational diseases began in earnest. As we came to understand the ways in which exposure to dusts, chemicals, vibration, noise and radiation could degrade human health, so we learnt how to implement effective strategies to prevent them from doing so. Largely it has been a story of spectacular success. Better understanding of industrial diseases, progressively more stringent health and safety legislation, and new technologies and automation have together decimated the toll of deaths and serious diseases associated with employment.

In the infancy of the twenty-first century, there are glimmers of where we are headed next. Amazon founder Jeff Bezos named his rocket company Blue Origin in recognition of how our planet appears when compared with the desolate, barren and inhospitable planets visualised by telescopes and unmanned spacecraft thus far: a blue marble in the inky blackness of space. As its unique beauty and suitability for human life become apparent, so we are reminded of its preciousness and the existential need to protect it. It is no coincidence that, as space exploration has become a reality over the course of the last couple of generations, so Green political parties, defined primarily by their concern for the environment, have emerged around the world.

To date, the debates about how economic growth and environmental concerns should be traded off against one another have been fairly parochial, Luddite and uninspiring. Bezos has advanced our thinking about the problem with his ability to see a somewhat bigger picture:[i] 'I think that over the next few hundred years we need to move our heavy industry off-planet. Our Earth will be zoned residential and light industrial. And that just makes a lot of sense! You shouldn't be doing heavy industry on Earth.'[1] Ultimately this will be the culmination of the collective efforts of all those who have striven to protect human health from the hazards of work. In the meantime, whilst astonishing progress has been made, the problem of industrial disease is diminishing in first-world countries not just because it is becoming smaller, but also because it is being displaced. Less mature economies are having their industrial revolutions now. The reality of globalised markets means that, where international corporates still need dangerous and dirty work to be done, it is liable to be offshored to jurisdictions with cheaper—meaning poorer—standards of health and safety regulation.

Given the exponential rate with which new technologies are emerging, we can be hopeful that we will complete the 200-year-old mission to minimise work's negative effect on health during the remainder of the twenty-first century. We will

---

[i] Professor Brian Cox, having interviewed Bezos for the BBC documentary *The 21st Century Race for Space*, stated: 'One of the worst ideas we've ever had in modern geopolitics is that we've got access to limited resources here on Earth, and it's false. If you think there's limited resources, then you compete for them. All you need to demonstrate is that you can get them elsewhere, in space.'

begin to displace industrial hazards not at the planetary scale, but on an interplanetary one. But we aspire to more: beyond jobs that do not kill, maim or impair quality of life, jobs that positively enhance people's sense of security, social inclusion and self-worth. Fortunately, this objective aligns with the needs of Western governments. Whilst work is an important contributor to health and is increasingly recognised as such, it is also the engine of our economy, and hence our prosperity and standard of living. Government and policy-makers are beginning to understand that advancing the cause of 'good work' is not just important ethically, as an end in its own right, nor just as a means of improving public health, but also as a means of optimising productivity.

Employers increasingly recognise how crucial employee engagement is, at least those organisations large enough to have a human resources department and to send their staff on training courses. As much as someone may have the potential to excel in their role, why should they bother to do more than the bare minimum if they don't care about their employer? Engagement is a major determinant of productivity, and hence the success, and sometimes the survival, of the organisation. Yet few employers have managed to earn impressive levels of engagement from their staff.[ii] It seems likely that the explanation for this is largely because, in the past, they didn't have to, and as times have changed they have simply been slow to adapt. The rot set in over the last 150 years, with industrialisation and the emergence of large corporates.

[ii] In its 2018 'UK Working Lives' report, the CIPD found that almost half of employees surveyed, 47%, did not feel that they were 'often' or 'always' enthusiastic about their work. Available at https://www.cipd. co.uk/Images/uk-working-lives-summary_tcm18–40233.pdf [Accessed 7 November 2018].

We might imagine that the gentler, softer skills of good management were probably more abundant in the preindustrial days when businesses were smaller, local, often family-run affairs. Then, the relationship between the worker and business-owner was direct—with the humanising quality that direct human contact brings—rather than through various management hierarchies. As the environment of work changed, as people became commoditised production units working anonymously within large factories, so the DNA encoding such emotional intelligence gradually disappeared from the management gene pool. This must have had a disenfranchising effect on production line workers and, as we have transitioned to a service-sector economy, the generation of office droids who followed them. But, until the mid 1990s, the labour market was fairly fluid: hiring, firing and resignations were a normal part of life rather than manna for legal melodrama. The manager who was not particularly creative in devising ways to make their team want to be in work could at least lazily resort to the fall-back threat of sacking them. Employees were motivated to attend work out of fear if not out of love.

As employment legislation has provided greater protections for employees, placing a greater premium on motivational than coercive leadership, the managers practising this particular style of employment relations have been found lacking. Now that the whip has been prised from their hand, they are more reliant on employees wanting to be in work, rather than feeling coerced into being there. It seems unlikely that managers will regain their whip-hand any time soon, at least until we hit an economic catastrophe so seismic that it creates a breach in the current dam of restrictive employment law. Instead, if there are to be more backsides on seats, and motivated backsides at that, managers are going to need to learn how to make their team's work more appealing. In the words of Studs Terkel, effective organisations should make work 'a daily search for meaning ... for recognition ... for astonishment ... a sort of life, rather than a Monday through Friday sort of dying.'

There are signs that the technological revolution in the workplace is beginning to facilitate this more aspirational approach to work in the UK. As the broadband infrastructure is upgraded—admittedly, much more slowly than in other parts of the world—internet speeds are accelerating. This, in conjunction with software that enables remote collaborative team working and videoconferencing, has freed many from the grind of commuting across a congested road and rail network. It has allowed them to live in areas where they feel their quality of life is likely to be highest, and not simply those in proximity to their workplace or to a transport hub. There are lingering management fears that employees who are not a permanent physical presence at headquarters will instead be on the school run, or gardening, or cripplingly dislocated from their team. But these seem to be dissipating as twenty-first-century ways of working become normalised, quite different from those of the twentieth century sweatshop. And, just as technology has facilitated home working, so it has enabled suspicious management to reassure themselves about the remote employee's productivity and performance in ways that they never could before. Real-time audit tools that assess the individual's output in quantitative terms can easily be embedded in the IT platforms used by different organisations. Even qualitative data is readily obtained. Client and customer perceptions of the work being produced are easily gauged by embedding feedback surveys in the company's communications and social media.

What's more, concerns about remoteness are easing as managers themselves begin to appreciate the convenience of videoconferencing. Virtual reality, and even holographic, conferencing technology is already in an advanced stage of development. The traditional assumption that teams of people can only work together when they are in physical proximity will seem progressively more outdated as time passes. Then there are the sizeable financial gains for employers who recognise the savings to be achieved by remote working. Most employers base their premises in fairly urban areas on the grounds that it is easier to recruit into places that are near to where people live, convenient for them to travel to, and with amenities within walking distance during lunch breaks. The ground rent on buildings in such areas comes at a cost. Decimating the square footage that is leased, as flexible working makes possible, can make a meaningful contribution to the company's efficiency and profitability.

The penny is even dropping amongst the more enlightened managers that, even if their staff are on the school run during working hours, or gardening, or—as a non-medical friend of mine has managed for some years—'working from the boat', this may not actually matter, if they are putting the hours in around these activities. Or even, provided that they are sufficiently productive—and managers now have the tools to assess that—if they are not doing the hours. The idea of remunerating someone according to the hours that they work is fairly anachronistic, a remnant from a time when shift length was as good a proxy measure for productivity as any other. It dates back to a period when many roles were mind-numbing and paced by a production line, where one worker's contribution per hour could really not be very different from another's. This is very different today.

It seems inherently fairer that people should be rewarded according to their contribution to an organisation, and not crudely in terms of the duration of their penal servitude towards it. Why should slower, less effective staff not have the opportunity to take on larger roles—otherwise denied to them—if the price is spending a greater proportion of their week than colleagues invested in their work? And why should the smart alecks not be free to practise their golf swing, or be at their children's mid-afternoon school concert, if they can satisfy the employer's expectation for the role in the hours that they are attending to their work? Flexible working is cheaper and massively widens the potential pool of talent from which the employer can recruit. But no account of the productivity gains to be achieved would be complete without coming back to that talisman of modern management theory: engagement. The modern epidemiological concern is that the frustration people feel within their straitjacket jobs is killing them off in droves; that micro-managing supervisors, who compel them to set about tasks in a prescriptive manner rather than in the way that comes most naturally to them, pose a mortal risk.[2] Whether or not this is true, there can be little doubt that most people are at least happier and better disposed to their employer when they are treated as adults. Engagement is inevitably higher amongst people who are given some latitude in how they work towards the employer's objectives. The manager's interactions with them are then perceived as supportive and helpful, an acknowledgement of the individual's ability to exercise their initiative and judgement, rather than as a crèche supervisor checking up on a wayward toddler. Most people will reciprocate this trust by working harder.

Employers seem more attuned to the fact that their employees do not want to feel like flagpole-sitters for the duration of their working life. There is an innate human need for satisfaction from work, for the individual to believe that what they are doing serves a purpose. If they see no tangible difference to the world around them as a result of their actions, and question the value of their job, this raises existential doubts about the importance of their own being as well. This was perhaps easier in a manufacturing economy where there was a physical product. Whilst the line worker might spend most of their time installing dashboards or brake discs, the physical manifestation of their efforts—and those of all the other workers—could at least be seen from time to time, by wandering across the factory to watch the finished product driving out under its own steam.

The various car manufacturers had a long tradition of holding on to vehicles with particular sentimental value, typically the last production example of a particular model, and for them to be signed across their paintwork by the hundreds of people who had spent years of their lives in the creation of these pieces of folded steel. At the British Motor Museum in Gaydon, a number of these exhibits are curated, recognisable to anyone growing up in the second half of the twentieth century. There is a 1946 Austin 16, signed by the Austin workforce to celebrate that it was the millionth car made by the company. Then there are a 1996 Austin/ Rover Montego and a 1998 Rover Metro, similarly signed, as the last of their kind. Workers felt it important to commemorate births too—the first Land Rover Freelander, from 1997, received this autographing treatment. It reveals something about the people who worked at these plants that they took the time to perform these symbolic acts, testament to what they had accomplished.

Companies in the service-sector economy have the more difficult task of attaching meaning to activities that do not result in a finished product that staff can touch and admire. Arguably they have the advantage that, though the product of their labours is intangible, their interactions with customers tend to be more immediate, with more potential for positive feedback—including through social media. However, the relatively high rates of turnover within UK call centres substantiates my impression that interacting repeatedly with the modern British consumer is frequently not especially gratifying.[iii] My experience is that service-

---

[iii] One consultancy has estimated turnover as being 75% higher than the UK average. Centralus (undated). 'Call Centre Turnover: A Vicious Circle

sector employers, too, are taking steps to help their employees appreciate the wider significance of their individual contribution. This might be through facilitating social networks of people working in different parts of the business, which allow different team members to talk to one another and express gratitude for the way the efforts of others enable them in their own roles. Similarly, there is more internal marketing to staff about the impact that the company's service has had on the lives of its customers, such as case studies about the way that prompt handling on an insurance claim has helped people in times of hardship.

One of the particular challenges that employers are already beginning to face is in finding ways to motivate people in jobs that can increasingly be done by computers. It has long been recognised that those jobs requiring consistent execution of algorithmic process are better performed by machines, but as each day passes it becomes clearer that things will not stop there. Those in more skilled roles, who were condescendingly sympathetic to their unskilled counterparts when the robot economy was first mooted, are becoming less complacent.[iv] The extraordinary capabilities of machine learning and artificial intelligence mean that many of these professional roles, where the premium may instead be on recognition of subtle patterns and the ability to exercise finely balanced judgement, are likely to become insecure too.

On inspecting a major construction site, William Aberhart thought it was absurd that men were toiling away with picks and shovels in a time when heavy plant was available—as ridiculous as

---

With No Easy Way Out'. Available at http://corporate.centralus.co.uk/articles/call-centre-turnover/ [Accessed 7 November 2018].

[iv] In the words of satirical 'demotivational' poster company Despair, Inc, 'The bad news is robots can do your job now. The good news is we're now hiring robot repair technicians. The worse news is we're working on robot-fixing robots—and we do not anticipate any further good news.'

expecting that they should excavate with knives and forks—simply to create work for them. What jobs will remain in the robot economy that will still make sense for a human to perform, without looking like exhibits in a working museum whilst doing so?

Presumably, those roles where there is some unique added value from human involvement. These are likely to be jobs where customers—and hence employers—attach particular importance to human contact, in a time when this may be an increasing rarity in commercial settings. This would be a reversal of the current trend for customer service to be delivered with as little human interaction as possible, evident in the proliferation of self-service checkouts and internet shopping. There are a number of reasons why, in a world where automation had been taken to a *Blade Runner*-style extreme, a premium might become reattached to human customer service. For richer customers, then as now, this might simply be a case of snobbery and a desire for exclusivity; for others, there might simply be a renewed appreciation for human contact once technological advances have made it sufficiently rare. There may also be some sectors where the value attached to human interaction is so inherent that it will never vanish—healthcare perhaps being a prime example.[v]

Different tiers of customer service may emerge, with the premium offering on both sides of the transaction being engage-

---

[v] Certainly within diagnostics the machines are coming. IBM's 'Watson' is a classic example: using 'big data' to develop profoundly insightful AI and applying it to machines that never tire, pattern recognition of X-ray interpretation has been revolutionised. Google has developed an algorithm that can predict heart disease from retinal scans showing blood vessels at the back of the eye. Some studies even suggest that acoustic speech analysis software may have promise in early detection of incipient heart failure. But who would want a computer or android to impart the news of such diagnosis, or discuss the risks and benefits of treatment with them?

ment with another human. The competition for this good work is likely to increase, as automation displaces many manual, low-skilled workers whilst also intruding into the lower-tier service roles. Selection forces will mean that only those with the desirable human skills of emotional intelligence, personability and even humour will fare well. Those without such attributes will be engaged in a race to the bottom, being underpriced by successive generations of progressively more efficient robots for the menial, physical jobs, or low-margin service jobs, that remain.

Worryingly, the evolution in technology seems to be outpacing our ability to adapt. The first generation of children to be born and raised after the dotcom boom will reach adulthood and begin looking for work over the next few years. They represent a vast social experiment as we assess to what extent very different methods of child-rearing—frequently involving the iPad nanny—have affected the development of this generation's communication abilities and soft skills.[3] This is occurring at exactly the moment in history when an aptitude for human interaction is going to be so vital to their prospects of securing meaningful work.

A tech executive once mused to me that his most worrying concern for the future was what the growing number of people finding themselves without work in this new economy might do. He is not alone in this fear, now an active source of debate. One difficult but rational conclusion is that a significant proportion of the population will become effectively unemployable, because they will lack the aptitude for any tasks that a robot cannot perform more cheaply and efficiently. This would be the realisation of the long-forecast dream—or nightmare—of a world where technology has liberated humankind from the obligation to work.

In Ancient Greece, work was not seen as having inherent virtue; it was a necessary evil, a punishment from Zeus, who had seen to it that nature no longer spontaneously produced food.

Greek aristocrats saw work as debasing and something to be done by slaves, whereas we see it as an important part of our identity and as a potential source of meaning in our lives. In the robot economy to come, the meaning and purpose of work will change again. The question is how we face this change; how should we choose to model and conceive work in a world where machines can do most jobs for us?

The productivity gains to be achieved through automation would give some scope to support a rump of the population that was not working, the much-vaunted 'citizen's income', whose time does seem to be approaching. Even so, there will be limits to what is sustainable. It may well be that the terms and conditions attached to such a lifestyle need to become stringent. Currently welfare supports procreation, with incremental increases in the amount of benefit paid to families choosing to have children whom, by their own efforts alone, they could not support. Presumably a system having to support so many people who are not in work would need to impose some kind of Malthusian limit, some means of controlling the number of hungry mouths to feed. This might necessitate a reversal of the existing rubric—for there to be a generous and comfortable citizen's income for those choosing to withdraw from productive life, but with incremental reductions in benefit for those among them having children. It may even be that society would decide that those not contributing to its prosperity should forfeit their right to have a say in how things are run—that they should lose their right to vote. Beveridge's ruminations from 1906 now seem, if anything, more likely to come to pass than they might have back then:

> Those men who through general defects are unable to fill such a whole place in industry, are to be recognised as 'unemployable'. They must become the acknowledged dependents of the State ... but with complete and permanent loss of all citizen rights—including not only the franchise but civil freedom and fatherhood.[4]

In any case, there seems a high risk of a dystopian future for many without careful forethought as to how we should organise a world with a substantial proportion of working-age people not working, as a fact of life in a robot economy. If society can adapt to such radical change, and find ways to resolve the political tensions that are likely to arise, what will the lives of those effectively excluded from employment be like if—as current evidence indicates—work is so fundamental to human health and wellbeing? We will likely need to revise our understanding of what 'work' means, to tease out those elements that are both health-giving and which exist independent of the need for task completion on behalf of an employer. The intention would then be to engineer these purposefully into a lifestyle that might come to revolutionise our entire concept of work itself: activity that is not remunerated, monotonous, dehumanising and doctrinaire, but instead social, interactive, variable, creative and self-determined.

Such a reappraisal of our humanity might prove to be our salvation, the more adapted belief system that I sense societies and cultures around the globe are striving to attain as age-old religious beliefs are supplanted by superficial technological experiences that ultimately leave us feeling more, not less, isolated from one another in a supposedly interconnected world. We may come to see that there is a third age for humankind: the first being a social phase where we lacked the benefits of industry, the second being an industrial phase where we lacked the benefits of society, and the third being a halcyon where we were finally able to enjoy both.

Futurology is fraught, and the endpoints I have suggested represent diametrically opposing visions of humanity. If we believe that it is in the gift of humans, and not computers, to be the masters of our own destiny, then this lends an urgency to the argument that we need to revolutionise the existing world of work where, for the moment, drudgery and money remain inescapable factors. If we can do this effectively, and transition our society such that the experience of work is at least more comfortable and bearable than is currently the case for many, we may increase the prospects of our longer-term transition being into the more optimistic version of the future. Otherwise, if we cannot escape work's connotations of misery and slavery, many may simply seize on the perceived opportunity to escape as and when it presents itself, into a paradigm of purposelessness and isolation that proves to be far worse.

Whatever may become of us, one thing is clear: employers will continue to experience endemic levels of sickness for as long as they remain so unimaginative and punitive in their thinking. In the words of one wise occupational physician, 'Employers get the absence they deserve.' They will increasingly need to invest effort in creating workplaces where people want to be rather than where they have to be, as work per se becomes increasingly optional among the remaining 'valuable' contributors. For their part, doctors, and occupational physicians in particular, can facilitate this change by not pandering to the desire of employers to commoditise wellness as something they can procure. Instead, doctors must help employers to see how much healthy workplaces and engaged employees are dependent on creating, from the ground up, a culture of trust and mutual self-interest between organisations and the people they employ.

How many policies and procedures of the modern employer have the exact opposite effect—of making it clear to employees that they are not trusted, and depicting a 'them-and-us' divide between managers and their teams? A colleague recounted to me a conversation he had had with a wise police inspector some years ago, at the end of a consultation. It was amazing, the inspector pointed out, how teenagers fresh out of the Metropolitan police academy could, on their first day of service, close a major road, call in the firearms team and the dog squad, or summon a police helicopter. He calculated that these pimply law enforcers could incur tens of thousands of pounds of cost within a matter of minutes. But, he wryly observed, look at the paperwork and bureaucracy that they would need to traverse in order to obtain a new pair of boots if their current ones were chafing. This would include the obligatory trip to the occupational health department to have the severity of their blisters documented for posterity.

Some employers have embraced the principle that it makes more sense to trust those they employ and rely on to deliver their service, than to infantilise and doubt them. A number of high-profile employers—typically those within the technology sector—have taken this to what some, currently, would consider an extreme. They have entirely dispensed with the idea of mandating a contractually set amount of time to be spent working, enabled by the emergence of new technology in monitoring and real-time connection. LinkedIn, Virgin Management and Eventbrite are all companies that do not set any limits on the annual leave entitlement of their staff;[5] nor does Netflix, which does not require approval of expense claims either.[6]

In organisations where a culture of trust and mutuality has developed to this extent, the idea of requiring employees to bring a note from their doctor before we accept their claim that they feel too ill to work must seem a vestige from the employment relations Stone Age. And, of course, it is.

NOTES

PREFACE

1. R.P.C. Handfield-Jones (1964). 'Who shall help the doctor? Ancillaries, prescriptions and certificates'. *Lancet* 284:7370 (1133–90).

1. MEASURING THE INDESCRIBABLE

1. J. Stuart Mill (1874). 'Essay V. On the Definition of Political Economy; and on the Method of Investigation Proper to it.', in *Essays on Some Unsettled Questions of Political Economy*, 2nd ed. London: Longmans, Green, Reader & Dyer, Essay V, paragraph 38. Available at https://archive.org/details/essaysonsomeunse00millrich [Accessed 3 May 2018].
2. Confederation of British Industry (2013). 'Fit for Purpose: Absence and Workplace Health Survey 2013'. Available at http://www.kmghp.com/assets/cbi-pfizer_absence___workplace_health_2013-(1).pdf [Accessed 16 October 2018].
3. Office for Budget Responsibility (2016). 'Welfare Trends Report: October 2016'. Available at http://budgetresponsibility.org.uk/docs/dlm_uploads/Welfare-Trends-Report.pdf [Accessed 5 November 2016].
4. NatCen Social Research (2013). 'British Social Attitudes 30'. Available at http://www.bsa.natcen.ac.uk/media/38723/bsa30_full_report_final.pdf [Accessed 6 November 2016].

2. TRENCH WARFARE

1. Department for Work and Pensions (2016). 'Annual Report and Accounts

2015–16'. Available at https://www.gov.uk/government/uploads/system/uploads/attachment_data/file/534933/dwp-annual-report-and-accounts-2015–2016.pdf [Accessed 5 November 2016]; HM Treasury (2016). 'Budget 2016'. Available at https://www.gov.uk/government/uploads/system/uploads/attachment_data/file/508193/HMT_Budget_2016_Web_Accessible.pdf [Accessed 5 November 2016].

2. Department for Work and Pensions (2016). 'Annual Report and Accounts 2015–16'. Available at https://www.gov.uk/government/uploads/system/uploads/attachment_data/file/534933/dwp-annual-report-and-accounts-2015–2016.pdf [Accessed 5 November 2016].

3. Office for Budget Responsibility (2016). 'Welfare Trends Report: October 2016'. Available at http://budgetresponsibility.org.uk/docs/dlm_uploads/Welfare-Trends-Report.pdf [Accessed 5 November 2016].

4. Office for Budget Responsibility (2016). 'Economic and Fiscal Outlook: March 2016'. Available at https://cdn.obr.uk/March2016EFO.pdf [Accessed 18 October 2018]; Office for Budget Responsibility (2018). 'Economic and Fiscal Outlook: October 2018'. Available at https://cdn.obr.uk/EFO_October–2018.pdf [Accessed 29 October 2018].

5. M. Bang Petersen et al. (2012). 'Who Deserves Help? Evolutionary Psychology, Social Emotions, and Public Opinion about Welfare'. *Political Psychology* 33(3): 395–418. Available at https://www.ncbi.nlm.nih.gov/pmc/articles/PMC3551585/#R22 [Accessed 19 November 2016].

6. L. Trotsky (1937). *The Revolution Betrayed*, p. 57. Available at https://archive.org/details/in.ernet.dli.2015.237974/page/n57 [Accessed 23 November 2018].

7. Section 10 of the Welfare Reform Act 2007.

8. Professor M. Harrington (2010). 'An Independent Review of the Work Capability Assessment'. The Stationery Office.

9. Professor M. Harrington (2012). 'An Independent Review of the Work Capability Assessment: Year Three'. The Stationery Office.

10. Dr P. Litchfield (2014). 'An Independent Review of the Work Capability Assessment: Year Five'. The Stationery Office. Available at https://www.gov.uk/government/uploads/system/uploads/attachment_data/file/380027/wca-fifth-independent-review.pdf [Accessed 5 November 2016].

3. TABLOID TALES

1. S. Linning (2014). 'Champion bodybuilder jailed for swindling £28,000 by claiming he was too ill to walk—even though he managed to win "Mr Wales" contest TWICE'. *Mail Online*, 3 November 2014. Available at http://www.dailymail.co.uk/news/article-2818786/Champion-body-builder-swindled-28-000-claiming-ill-walk-managed-win-Mr-Wales-contest-TWICE.html [Accessed 6 November 2016].
2. R. Pocklington and A. Glendinning (2014). 'See kung fu benefit cheat who pocketed £35,000 in Disability Allowance despite teaching martial arts and Ju-Jitsu'. *The Mirror*, 22 February 2014. Available at http://www.mirror.co.uk/news/uk-news/see-kung-fu-benefit-cheat-3172888 [Accessed 6 November 2016].
3. R. Kennedy (2014). 'Benefit cheat who claimed he could not walk 10 yards caught playing 18 holes of golf'. *The Mirror*, 13 November 2014. Available at http://www.mirror.co.uk/news/uk-news/benefit-cheat-who-claimed-could-4624593 [Accessed 6 November 2016].
4. R. Smith (2014). '"Bed bound" benefits cheat caught after holiday snaps showed him ON A JET SKI'. *The Mirror*, 26 August 2014. Available at http://www.mirror.co.uk/news/uk-news/bed-bound-benefits-cheat-caught-4108822 [Accessed 6 November 2016].
5. *Sunday Express* (2014). 'Benefits cheat "too scared to leave house" jailed after being spotted on beach in INDIA'. 25 July 2014. Available at http://www.express.co.uk/news/uk/491947/Agoraphobic-benefits-cheat-jailed-after-being-spotted-on-beach-in [Accessed 6 November 2016].
6. *The Telegraph* (2010). '"Wheelchair-bound" benefits cheat caught dancing'. 4 August 2010. Available at http://www.telegraph.co.uk/news/newsvideo/7926461/Wheelchair-bound-benefits-cheat-caught-dancing.html [Accessed 6 November 2016].
7. L. Traynor (21 August 2014). 'Town mayor who pocketed £13,000 in disability benefits caught marching over a MILE during parade'. *The Mirror*, 21 August 2014. Available at http://www.mirror.co.uk/news/uk-news/town-mayor-who-pocketed-13000-4086865 [Accessed 6 November 2016].
8. N. Britten (2010). 'Football referee mayor claimed disability benefit'.

The Telegraph, 4 August 2010. Available at http://www.telegraph.co.uk/news/1896614/Football-referee-mayor-claimed-disability-benefit.html [Accessed 6 November 2016].

9. H. Clare (2017). 'Benefits cheat claimed she was too disabled to walk a metre is caught out by holiday snaps where she's snorkelling'. *The Mirror*, 31 July 2017. Available at http://www.mirror.co.uk/news/uk-news/benefits-cheat-claimed-disabled-walk-10906051 [Accessed 3 August 2017].

10. *The Telegraph* (2017). 'Benefits cheat paratrooper who claimed he was too weak to walk 50m caught out climbing Kilimanjaro'. 20 July 2017. Available at http://www.telegraph.co.uk/news/2017/07/20/benefits-cheat-paratrooper-claimed-weak-walk-50m-caught-climbing/ [Accessed 3 August 2017].

11. L. Keay (2018). 'Disability fraudster, 70, whose benefits fraud investigator wife helped him scam £20,000 by stating he could only walk 60 yards is spared jail... despite being filmed on a ZIP WIRE'. *The Daily Mail*, 27 September 2018. Available at: https://www.dailymail.co.uk/news/article-6213567/Clacton-fraudster-Paul-Stevens-DWP-wife-Alexandra-spared-jail-20-000-fraud.html [Accessed 7 October 2018].

12. F. Ryan (2016). 'The phantom benefit cheat is the perfect patsy for austerity'. *The Guardian*, 8 March 2016. Available at: https://www.theguardian.com/society/commentisfree/2016/mar/08/phantom-benefit-cheat-austerity-fraud-hotline [Accessed 21 April 2018].

13. YouGov UK (2015). 'One in five workers has pulled a sickie this year'. 27 October 2015. Available at: https://yougov.co.uk/news/2015/10/27/one-five-workers-have-pulled-sickie-year/ [Accessed 6 November 2016].

14. This was a poll entitled 'The Effects of a Sick Day', admittedly carried out on behalf of a yoghurt drink manufacturer rather than a more august institution. Nevertheless it adds to the polling data that suggests low-level malingering is something of an endemic phenomenon. Figures reported in 'One Third of Naughty Brits Have Pulled a "Sickie" Off Work This Year', PR Newswire, 27 October 2015. Available at http://www.prnewswire.co.uk/news-releases/one-third-of-naughty-

brits-have-pulled-a-sickie-off-work-this-year-537290591.html [Accessed 30 October 2018].

15. Ceridian (2006). 'Health in the Workplace: October 2006', p. 18. Available at http://docplayer.net/8461493-Health-in-the-workplace. html [Accessed 19 November 2016].

16. National Highway Traffic Safety Administration (2011). '2011 National Survey of Speeding Attitudes and Behaviors'. Available at https://www. nhtsa.gov/sites/nhtsa.dot.gov/files/2011_n_survey_of_speeding_attitudes_and_behaviors_811865.pdf [Accessed 24 September 2017].

17. NatCen Social Research (2013). 'British Social Attitudes 30'. Available at http://www.bsa.natcen.ac.uk/media/38723/bsa30_full_report_final. pdf [Accessed 6 November 2016].

18. The Stationery Office (2008). 'Working for a Healthier Tomorrow: Dame Carol Black's Review of the Health of Britain's Working Age Population'. Available at https://www.gov.uk/government/uploads/ system/uploads/attachment_data/file/209782/hwwb-working-for-a-healthier-tomorrow.pdf [Accessed 5 November 2016]; The Stationery Office (2011). 'Health at Work: An Independent Review of Sickness Absence'. Available at https://www.gov.uk/government/uploads/system/uploads/attachment_data/file/181060/health-at-work.pdf [Accessed 5 November 2016]; G. Waddell, K. Burton, N. Kendall (2008). 'Vocational Rehabilitation: What works, for whom, and when?'. University of Huddersfield, evidence statement MH-12, p. 23. Available at http://eprints.hud.ac.uk/id/eprint/5575/1/waddellburtonkendall2008-VR.pdf [Accessed 26 September 2017].

19. Department for Work and Pensions (2016). 'Annual Report and Accounts 2015–16'. Available at https://www.gov.uk/government/ uploads/system/uploads/attachment_data/file/534933/dwp-annual-report-and-accounts-2015–2016.pdf [Accessed 5 November 2016].

20. Department for Work and Pensions (2016). 'Fraud and Error in the Benefit System: Preliminary Data for 2015/16'. Available at https:// www.gov.uk/government/uploads/system/uploads/attachment_data/ file/528719/fraud-and-error-prelim-estimates-2015–16.pdf [Accessed 7 November 2016].

21. *The Telegraph* (2010). '"Wheelchair-bound" benefits cheat caught danc-

ing'; Pocklington and Glendinning (2014). 'See kung fu benefit cheat who pocketed £35,000 in Disability Allowance despite teaching martial arts and Ju-Jitsu'.

4. A TWO-WAY STREET

1. Sir William Beveridge (1942). 'Social insurance and allied services: Report by Sir William Beveridge'. London, HMSO. Available at https://archive.org/details/in.ernet.dli.2015.275849 [Accessed 3 May 2018].
2. Ibid., p. 6.
3. Ibid., p. 7.
4. W. Beveridge (1906). 'The Problem of the Unemployed'. *The Sociological Review* 3:1, 323–41. Available at http://journals.sagepub.com/doi/pdf/10.1177/0038026106SP300130.
5. Sir William Beveridge (1942). 'Social insurance and allied services', p. 58.
6. University of Bristol (2008). 'Press release: Fair rules for welfare reforms'. Available at http://www.bristol.ac.uk/news/2008/6040.html [Accessed 12 November 2016].
7. Andrew Marr (2007). *A History of Modern Britain*, p. 62. London: Macmillan.
8. *Hansard* (1944). HC Deb., vol. 396, col. 1780W (9 February 1944). 'Beveridge Report (sales)'. Available at https://api.parliament.uk/historic-hansard/written-answers/1944/feb/09/beveridge-report-sales [Accessed 3 May 2018].
9. D. Boyle (2014). 'Why Britain bombed Germany with copies of the Beveridge report: Dream of a welfare state "helped bring down Hitler"'. *Mail Online*, 23 May 2014. Available at http://www.dailymail.co.uk/news/article-2637305/The-dream-welfare-state-helped-bring-Hitler-How-British-airmen-dropped-copies-social-security-report-Europe-sparking-hopes-better-future-without-Nazis.html#ixzz4Ppp9Qoqe [Accessed 12 November 2016].
10. BBC News Online (2012). 'Beveridge report: from "deserving poor" to "scroungers"?' 26 November 2012. Available at http://www.bbc.co.uk/news/magazine-20431729 [Accessed 12 November 2016].

11. The Stationery Office (2008). 'Working for a Healthier Tomorrow: Dame Carol Black's Review of the Health of Britain's Working Age Population'. Available at https://www.gov.uk/government/uploads/system/uploads/attachment_data/file/209782/hwwb-working-for-a-healthier-tomorrow.pdf [Accessed 5 November 2016]; The Stationery Office (2011). 'Health at Work: An Independent Review of Sickness Absence'. Available at https://www.gov.uk/government/uploads/system/uploads/attachment_data/file/181060/health-at-work.pdf [Accessed 5 November 2016].

12. HMG (2015). 'Government to increase support for benefit claimants with addictions and treatable conditions'. Press release, 29 July 2015. Available at https://www.gov.uk/government/news/government-to-increase-support-for-benefit-claimants-with-addictions-and-treatable-conditions [Accessed 5 November 2016].

13. S. Hawkes (2015). 'Fat's all folks—Handout Brits told to lose flab or lose benefits'. *The Sun*, 28 July 2015. Available at https://www.thesun.co.uk/archives/politics/115493/fats-all-folks/ [Accessed 5 November 2016].

14. S. Wessely and G. Smith (2015). 'Linking benefits to treatment is unethical, and probably illegal'. *The Guardian*, 29 July 2015. Available at https://www.theguardian.com/commentisfree/2015/jul/29/coercing-people-mental-health-problems-work-treatment [Accessed 5 November 2016].

15. BBC Radio 4 (2015). *The Life Scientific: Dame Carol Black*. 6 October 2015. Available at https://www.bbc.co.uk/programmes/b06flmbf [Accessed 3 May 2018]; BBC Radio 4 (2016). 'Professor Dame Carol Black', *Desert Island Discs*. 12 February 2016. Available at https://www.bbc.co.uk/programmes/b06zqchz [Accessed 3 May 2018].

16. The Stationery Office (2016). 'An Independent Review into the impact on employment outcomes of drug or alcohol addiction, and obesity'. Available at https://www.gov.uk/government/uploads/system/uploads/attachment_data/file/573891/employment-outcomes-of-drug-or-alcohol-addiction-and-obesity.pdf [Accessed 16 May 2017].

17. Ibid., Executive Summary, para. 46, p. 14.

18. The Employment and Support Allowance Regulations 2008, Regulation

35(2)b. Available at http://www.legislation.gov.uk/uksi/2008/794/reg-ulation/35/made [Accessed 3 May 2018].

19. B. Barr et al. (2015). '"First, do no harm": are disability assessments associated with adverse trends in mental health? A longitudinal eco-logical study'. *Journal of Epidemiology and Community Health* 70 (1–7). Available at http://jech.bmj.com/content/early/2015/10/26/jech-2015-206209.full.pdf+html [Accessed 15 November 2016].

20. P. Butler and J. Pring (2016). 'Suicides of benefit claimants reveal DWP flaws, says inquiry'. *The Guardian* 13 May 2016. Available at https://www.theguardian.com/society/2016/may/13/suicides-of-benefit-claimants-reveal-dwp-flaws-says-inquiry [Accessed 15 November 2016]; A. Gentleman (2014). 'Vulnerable man starved to death after benefits were cut'. *The Guardian* 28 February 2014. Available at https://www.theguardian.com/society/2014/feb/28/man-starved-to-death-after-benefits-cut [Accessed 15 November 2016].

21. L. Traynor (2013). 'Benefit cuts blind man committed suicide after Atos ruled him fit to work'. *The Mirror*, 28 December 2013. Available at http://www.mirror.co.uk/news/uk-news/benefit-cuts-blind-man-committed-2965375 [Accessed 15 November 2016].

22. *The Huffington Post* (2013). 'Atos Benefits Row: Transplant Patient Linda Wootton Dies After Being Judged "Fit For Work"'. 28 May 2013. Available at http://www.huffingtonpost.co.uk/2013/05/28/linda-wootton-dies-after-being-judged-fit-for-work_n_3346582.html [Accessed 15 November 2016].

23. L. Crossley (2015). 'Coroner rules man with severe mental illness killed himself after he was found to be "fit to work" in a government assess-ment and lost access to his disability benefits'. *Mail Online*, 21 September 2015. Available at http://www.dailymail.co.uk/news/arti-cle-3243043/Coroner-rules-man-severe-mental-illness-killed-fit-work-government-assessment-lost-access-disability-benefits.html [Accessed 15 November 2016].

24. C. McDonald (2013). 'Heartbroken dad blames benefits axemen for driving his ill son to commit suicide'. *Daily Record*, 22 September 2013. Available at http://www.dailyrecord.co.uk/news/scottish-news/heart-

broken-dad-blames-benefits-axemen-2292176 [Accessed 15 November 2016].

25. National Audit Office (2016). 'Contracted-out health and disability assessments'. 8 January 2016. Available at https://www.nao.org.uk/wp-content/uploads/2016/01/Contracted-out-health-and-disability-assessments-Summary.pdf [Accessed 15 November 2016].

26. Dr Paul Litchfield (2014). 'An Independent Review of the Work Capability Assessment: Year Five'. The Stationery Office. Available at https://www.gov.uk/government/uploads/system/uploads/attachment_data/file/380027/wca-fifth-independent-review.pdf [Accessed 5 November 2016]. The report expresses surprise that twice as many applicants were being awarded higher-tier benefits through Regulation 35(2)(b) than in the preceding year. He speculated a number of reasons why this might be, but not the fact that various websites that help to coach applicants in completing their applications were campaigning, disingenuously or not, to raise awareness of Regulation 35.

27. Andrew Malleson (1973). *The Medical Run-Around*, p. 205. New York: Hart.

5. DOCTOR PRIESTS

1. The Charities Aid Foundation estimated that £10.1 billion was donated to charities within the UK in 2015. In the same year, DWP spending was £173 billion. Charities Aid Foundation (2016). 'An overview of charitable giving in the UK during 2015'. Available at https://www.cafonline.org/docs/default-source/personal-giving/caf_ukgiving2015_1891a_web_230516.pdf [Accessed 29 October 2018]; Department for Work and Pensions (2016). 'Annual Report and Accounts 2015–16'. Available at https://www.gov.uk/government/uploads/system/uploads/attachment_data/file/534933/dwp-annual-report-and-accounts-2015-2016.pdf [Accessed 5 November 2016].

2. Ivan Illich (1976). *Limits to Medicine*, p. 71. New York: Bantam.

3. A. Hall (2017). 'Germany Green Party pledges to pay for free sex with prostitutes for anyone who needs "sexual assistance" and can't afford it'. *The Daily Mail*, 9 January 2017. Available at: http://www.dailymail.co.uk/news/article-4101376/Sex-prostitutes-paid-Government-needs-

sexual-assistance-afford-hooker-German-Green-Party-plans.html [Accessed 13 January 2017].

4. *The Irish Times* (2018). 'Doctor under fire for note freeing woman from gym membership'. 17 April 2018. Available at https://www.irishtimes.com/news/offbeat/doctor-under-fire-for-note-freeing-woman-from-gym-membership-1.3464831 [Accessed 21 April 2018].

5. L. Bever and E. Rosenberg (2018). 'United changed its policy for emotional-support animals. That peacock still can't board.' *The Washington Post*, 1 February 2018. Available at https://www.washingtonpost.com/news/animalia/wp/2018/01/30/a-woman-tried-to-board-a-plane-with-her-emotional-support-peacock-united-wouldnt-let-it-fly/?noredirect=on&utm_term=.faa40fb4f83a [Accessed 22 April 2018].

6. N. Khomami (2017). 'Construction firm Mears bans workers from having beards'. *The Guardian*, 1 June 2017. Available at https://www.theguardian.com/business/2017/jun/01/construction-firm-mears-bans-workers-from-having-beards [Accessed 22 April 2018].

7. M. McLuhan (1964). 'Chapter 1: The Medium is the Message', in *Understanding Media: The Extensions of Man*. New York: McGraw-Hill. Available at http://web.mit.edu/allanmc/www/mcluhan.mediummessage.pdf [Accessed 22 April 2018].

8. E. J. Ingebretsen (1982). 'The Priestly Ministry of the Doctor'. *The Linacre Quarterly* 49:3, Article 4. Available at http://epublications.marquette.edu/lnq/vol49/iss3/4 [Accessed 13 November 2016]. Ingebretsen's piece is a good example of the form; *The Linacre Quarterly* itself is the journal of the Catholic Medical Association.

9. I. Illich (1976). *Limits to Medicine*, p. 79.

6. SICK-NOTES

1. O. Clarke (1912). *The National Insurance Act 1911: Being a treatise on the scheme of the National Health Insurance and Insurance against Unemployment created by that Act, with the encorporated enactments, full explanatory notes, tables and examples*. London: Butterworth & Co. Available at https://archive.org/details/nationalinsuranc00clar [Accessed 4 April 2018].

2. C. Schuster (1914). 'Report of the Departmental Committee on

sickness benefit claims under the National Insurance Act. Cd. 7687. National Health Insurance. London: HM Stationery Office. Available at https://archive.org/details/b21361125_001 [Accessed 4 May 2018].
3. Ibid., p. 37.
4. J. Gulland (2011). '"Excessive sickness claims": controlling sickness and incapacity benefits in the early 20th century'. Paper presented to the Social Policy Association annual conference, Lincoln. Available at http://www.social-policy.org.uk/lincoln2011/Gulland%20P6.pdf [Accessed 13 November 2016].
5. W. Beveridge (1906). 'The Problem of the Unemployed'. *The Sociological Review* 3:1 (323–41). Available at http://journals.sagepub.com/doi/pdf/10.1177/0038026106SP300130 [Accessed 3 May 2018].
6. L. Byrne (2012). 'Speech: Britain's New Bargain: Social Security For One Nation Britain'. 1 December 2012. Available at http://liambyrne.co.uk/research_archive/britains-new-bargain-social-security-for-one-nation-britain-my-speech-to-the-fabian-society-on-the-70th-anniversary-of-the-beveridge-report-1st-december-2012-toynbee-hall/ [Accessed 25 November 2017].
7. P. Addison (1975). *The Road to 1945*, p. 117. London: Jonathan Cape.
8. K. Martin (1963). 'Obituary: William Beveridge (1879–1963)'. *New Statesman*, 22 March 1963, edited & reprinted 30 November 2012. Available at https://www.newstatesman.com/2012/11/obituary-william-beveridge-1879-1963 [Accessed 25 November 2017].
9. HMG (1948). 'National Health Service: Attitude of the medical profession'. Cabinet Paper 23, Memorandum by Aneurin Bevan, Minister of Health. Available at http://filestore.nationalarchives.gov.uk/pdfs/small/cab-129-23-cp-23.pdf [Accessed 13 November 2016].
10. British Medical Association (1948). 'Doctors' poll on NHS'. 19 February 1948. Available at http://www.nationalarchives.gov.uk/pathways/citizenship/brave_new_world/transcripts/plebiscite.htm [Accessed 13 November 2016].
11. British Medical Association (1946). 'British Medical Association and the National Health Service Bill'. Available at http://contentdm.warwick.ac.uk/cdm/ref/collection/health/id/1617 [Accessed 13 November 2016].

7. PARADISE LOST

1. National Joint Registry for England, Wales, Northern Ireland and the Isle of Man (2016). '13th Annual Report'. Available at http://www.njr-reports.org.uk/Portals/0/PDFdownloads/NJR%2013th%20Annual%20Report%202016.pdf [Accessed 30 July 2017]. This identifies 796,636 surviving patients with artificial hips, for a population size of 60,243,400 people (ONS figures for the UK population size in 2016, excluding Scotland which the NJR statistics do not include).

2. J. E. Powell (1962). 'Lloyd Roberts Lecture: Health and Wealth'. *Proceedings of the Royal Society of Medicine* 55 (1–6). Available at https://www.ncbi.nlm.nih.gov/pmc/articles/PMC1896398/pdf/procrsmed00237–0006.pdf [Accessed 10 November 2016].

3. Professor J. N. Morris (1965). 'Capacity and Incapacity for Work: Some Recent History'. *Proceedings of the Royal Society of Medicine* 58 (821–5). Available at https://www.ncbi.nlm.nih.gov/pmc/articles/PMC1898948/pdf/procrsmed00191–0076.pdf [Accessed 10 November 2016].

4. P J Taylor (1967). 'Individual variations in sickness absence'. *British Journal of Industrial Medicine* 24 (169–77). Available at http://oem.bmj.com/content/24/3/169.full.pdf+html [Accessed 10 November 2016].

5. T. Burchardt (1999). 'The Evolution of Disability Benefits in the UK: Re-weighting the basket'. Available at Centre for Analysis of Social Exclusion: http://eprints.lse.ac.uk/6490/1/The_Evolution_of_Disability_Benefits_in_the_UK_Re-weighting_the_basket.pdf [Accessed 13 November 2016].

6. M. Levinson (2017). *An Extraordinary Time: The End of the Postwar Boom and the Return of the Ordinary Economy*, pp. 196–7. London: Random House.

7. N. Watt (2015). 'Osborne distances himself from Thatcher legacy over disability benefits'. *The Guardian*, 29 July 2015. Available at https://www.theguardian.com/politics/2013/apr/02/osborne-thatcher-legacy-disability-benefits [Accessed 10 November 2016]; Tony Blair (2010). *A Journey: My Political Life*, p. 210. Toronto: Knopf Canada. Former Prime Minister Tony Blair included the following nugget in his memoirs: 'We talked of the dramatic reduction in the numbers of unemployed, but

this masked the huge rise in numbers on incapacity benefit that had taken place under the Tories and was continuing under us, and the Green Paper proposed only tinkering changes in this crucial area.'

8. G. Waddell and A. K. Burton (2006). 'Is work good for your health and well-being?' London: The Stationery Office. Available at https:// www.gov.uk/government/uploads/system/uploads/attachment_data/ file/214326/hwwb-is-work-good-for-you.pdf [Accessed 31 July 2017].
9. Department of Health (2004). 'Choosing health: making healthy choices easier', Chapter 7 'Work and Health', p. 156. Available at http:// webarchive.nationalarchives.gov.uk/+/http://www.dh.gov.uk/en/ Publicationsandstatistics/Publications/PublicationsPolicyAnd Guidance/DH_4094550 [Accessed 24 September 2018].
10. HMG (2005). 'Health, work and wellbeing: caring for our future. A strategy for the health and wellbeing of working age people', p. 19. Available at https://assets.publishing.service.gov.uk/government/ uploads/system/uploads/attachment_data/file/209570/health-and-well-being.pdf [Accessed 24 September 2018].
11. F. E. Whitehead (1972). 'Recent Trends in Certificated Sickness Absence'. *Proceedings of the Royal Society of Medicine* 65 (567–72). Available at https://www.ncbi.nlm.nih.gov/pmc/articles/PMC1643947/ pdf/procrsmed00346–0087.pdf [Accessed 13 November 2016]; J. Banks, R. Blundell and C. Emmerson (2015). 'Disability Benefit Receipt and Reform: Reconciling Trends in the United Kingdom'. *Journal of Economic Perspectives* 29:2 (173–90). Available at http://pubs.aeaweb. org/doi/pdfplus/10.1257/jep.29.2.173 [Accessed 13 November 2016].
12. Banks, Blundell and Emmerson (2015). 'Disability Benefit Receipt and Reform'.
13. *Hansard* (1993). Hansard, HC Deb., vol. 226, col. 732 (15 June 1993). Available at https://api.parliament.uk/historic-hansard/commons/1993/ jun/15/engagements [Accessed 4 May 2018].
14. Welfare Reform Act 2007. Available at http://www.legislation.gov.uk/ ukpga/2007/5/part/1/crossheading/assessments-relating-to-entitle-ment [Accessed 14 November 2016].
15. Department for Work and Pensions (2010). 'Universal Credit: Welfare that Works'. Available at https://www.gov.uk/government/uploads/

system/uploads/attachment_data/file/181145/universal-credit-full-document.pdf [Accessed 14 November 2016].

16. Office for Budget Responsibility (2016). 'Welfare Trends Report: October 2016'. Available at http://budgetresponsibility.org.uk/docs/dlm_uploads/Welfare-Trends-Report.pdf [Accessed 5 November 2016].

17. ONS (2014). 'Sickness absence in the labour market: February 2014'. Available at http://www.ons.gov.uk/employmentandlabourmarket/peopleinwork/labourproductivity/articles/sicknessabsenceinthelabourmarket/2014–02–25 [Accessed 16 November 2016]; CBI (2013). 'Fit for purpose: Absence and workplace health survey 2013'. Available at http://www.kmghp.com/assets/cbi-pfizer_absence___workplace_health_2013-(1).pdf [Accessed 18 October 2018].

18. ONS (2016). 'Sickness absence in the labour market: February 2016'. Available at https://www.ons.gov.uk/employmentandlabourmarket/peopleinwork/labourproductivity/articles/sicknessabsenceinthelabourmarket/2016 [Accessed 26 November 2017].

8. DISEASE INSPECTORS

1. A. J. Cronin (1939). *The Citadel*. London: Victor Gollancz. Available at https://archive.org/details/in.ernet.dli.2015.527636 [Accessed 4 May 2018].

2. S O'Mahony (2012). 'A. J. Cronin and *The Citadel*: did a work of fiction contribute to the foundation of the NHS?' *Journal of the Royal College of Physicians of Edinburgh* 42 (172–8S). Available at https://www.rcpe.ac.uk/sites/default/files/omahony_0.pdf [Accessed 24 September 2018].

3. Cronin (1939). *The Citadel*, p. 135.

4. Ibid., p. 135.

5. Ibid., p. 136.

6. Ibid., p. 137.

7. A. J. Cronin (1952). *Adventures in Two Worlds*, p. 89. London: Victor Gollancz.

8. A. Smith (2016). 'Post-truth politics is a myth: this is the post-trust era'. *Politics*, 21 November 2016. Available at http://www.politics.co.uk/comment-analysis/2016/11/21/post-truth-politics-is-a-myth-this-is-a-post-trust-era [Accessed 28 April 2018].

9. S. Boseley (2017). 'NHS workers urged to be alert for sepsis and treat within an hour'. *The Guardian*, 10 March 2017. Available at https://www.theguardian.com/society/2017/mar/10/nhs-workers-urged-be-alert-for-sepsis-and-treat-within-an-hour [Accessed 27 April 2018]; PA (2017). 'Don't ask GPs for antibiotics, new health campaign urges'. *The Guardian*, 23 October 2017. Available at https://www.theguardian.com/society/2017/oct/23/dont-ask-gps-for-antibiotics-new-health-campaign-urges [Accessed 27 April 2018].

10. Professor J. N. Morris (1965). 'Capacity and Incapacity for Work: Some Recent History'. *Proceedings of the Royal Society of Medicine* 58 (821–5). Available at https://www.ncbi.nlm.nih.gov/pmc/articles/PMC1898948/pdf/procrsmed00191–0076.pdf [Accessed 10 November 2016].

11. R. V. Sires (1955). 'Labor Unrest in England, 1910–1914'. *The Journal of Economic History* 15:3 (246–66).

12. A. Malleson (1973). *The Medical Run-Around*, p. 196. New York: Hart.

13. Morris (1965). 'Capacity and Incapacity for Work'.

14. H. H. Bashford (1944). Some Aspects of Sikness Absence in Industry. *British Journal of Industrial Medicine* 1:1 (7–10). Available at https://www.ncbi.nlm.nih.gov/pmc/articles/PMC1035553/pdf/brjindmed00269–0011.pdf [Accessed 7 October 2018].

9. RELUCTANT GAMEKEEPERS

1. M. Haberman and L. K. Altman (2015). 'Donald Trump Releases Medical Report Calling His Health "Extraordinary"'. *The New York Times*, 14 December 2015. Available at https://www.nytimes.com/politics/first-draft/2015/12/14/donald-trump-releases-medical-report-calling-his-health-extraordinary/ [Accessed 2 May 2018].

2. L. K. Altman (2017). 'Donald Trump's Longtime Doctor Says President Takes Hair-Growth Drug'. *The New York Times*, 1 February 2017. Available at https://www.nytimes.com/2017/02/01/us/politics/trump-prostate-drug-hair-harold-bornstein.html [Accessed 2 May 2018].

3. D. Reid (2018). 'Trump wrote his own "astonishingly excellent" health letter, claims former doctor'. CNBC, 2 May 2018. Available at https://www.cnbc.com/2018/05/02/trump-wrote-his-own-doctors-health-letter-claim-made.html [Accessed 2 May 2018]; CNN Politics (2018).

'Exclusive: Bornstein claims Trump dictated the glowing health letter'. 2 May 2018. Available at https://edition.cnn.com/2018/05/01/politics/harold-bornstein-trump-letter/index.html [Accessed 2 May 2018]; NBC News (2018). 'Trump doctor Harold Bornstein says bodyguard, lawyer "raided" his office, took medical files'. 1 May 2018. Available at https://www.nbcnews.com/politics/donald-trump/trump-doc-says-trump-bodyguard-lawyer-raided-his-office-took-n870351 [Accessed 2 May 2018].

4. CBC News Canada (1998). 'Manitoba doctors face "blue flu" fines'. 4 December 1998. Available at http://www.cbc.ca/news/canada/manitoba-doctors-face-blue-flu-fines-1.166006 [Accessed 16 November 2016].

5. S. Hussey et al. (2003). 'Sickness certification system in the United Kingdom: qualitative study of views of general practitioners in Scotland'. *British Medical Journal*, 22 December 2003. Available at http://www.bmj.com/content/bmj/328/7431/88.full.pdf [Accessed 16 November 2016].

6. General Medical Council (2013). 'Good medical practice. Domain 3: Communication, partnership and teamwork—Establish and maintain partnerships with patients', paras 46–52. Available at http://www.gmc-uk.org/guidance/good_medical_practice/partnerships.asp [Accessed 19 November 2016]; Royal College of General Practitioners (2016). 'Continuity of care in modern day general practice'. Available to download from http://www.rcgp.org.uk/policy/rcgp-policy-areas/continuity-of-care.aspx [Accessed 19 November 2016].

7. S. Hussey et al. (2003). 'Sickness certification system in the United Kingdom'.

8. J. Elms et al. (2005). 'The perceptions of occupational health in primary care'. *Occupational Medicine*, 1 September 2005. Available at https://academic.oup.com/occmed/article/55/7/523/1421931 [Accessed 16 November 2016].

9. *Forbes* (2015). 'The world's biggest employers (infographic)'. 23 June 2015. Available at http://www.forbes.com/sites/niallmccarthy/2015/06/23/the-worlds-biggest-employers-infographic/#41b1451b51d0 [Accessed 16 November 2016].

10. H. T. O. Davies, C. Hodges and T. G. Rundall (2003). 'Views of doctors and managers on the doctor-manager relationship in the NHS'. *British Medical Journal*, 22 March 2003. Available at http://www.bmj.com/content/bmj/326/7390/626.full.pdf [Accessed 16 November 2016]; R. Agius et al. (1996). 'Survey of perceived stress and work demands of consultant doctors'. *Occupational and Environmental Medicine* 53 (217–24). Available at http://oem.bmj.com/content/53/4/217.full.pdf+html [Accessed 19 November 2016]; S. Boorman (2009). 'NHS health and wellbeing review: interim report'. Department of Health. Available at http://webarchive.nationalarchives.gov.uk/20130107105354/http://www.dh.gov.uk/prod_consum_dh/groups/dh_digitalassets/documents/digitalasset/dh_108910.pdf [Accessed 19 November 2016]. While three-quarters of NHS chief executives are satisfied with the power balance between managers and doctors, this drops to fewer than half of clinical directors; neither managers nor doctors feel that there are adequate resources; and only 38 per cent of clinical directors think that management is generally responsive to resource requests to correct this.

11. R. Mulholland (2017). 'French doctor reprimanded for signing off 4,200 sick days in just four months'. *The Telegraph*, 29 June 2017. Available at http://www.telegraph.co.uk/news/2017/06/29/french-doctor-reprimanded-signing-4200-sick-days-just-four-months/ [Accessed 6 August 2017].

12. R. Roope, G. Parker and S. Turner (2009). 'General practitioners' use of sickness certificates'. *Occupational Medicine* 59 (580–85). Available at https://academic.oup.com/occmed/article/59/8/580/1371098 [Accessed 17 November 2016].

13. J. Elms et al. (2005). 'The perceptions of occupational health in primary care'.

14. N. Elmore et al. (2016). 'Investigating the relationship between consultation length and patient experience: a cross-sectional study in primary care'. *British Journal of General Practice*, 25 October 2016. Available at http://bjgp.org/content/carly/2016/10/24/bjgp16X687733/tab-pdf [Accessed 19 November 2016].

15. G. Irving et al. (2017). 'International variations in primary care phy-

sician consultation time: a systematic review of 67 countries'. *BMJ Open*, 8 November 2017. Available at http://bmjopen.bmj.com/content/7/10/e017902#T1 [Accessed 9 November 2017].

16. Australian Broadcasting Corporation (2011). 'Health Report: Ganfyd— the sick saga of sickness certificates'. 5 December 2011. Available at http://www.abc.net.au/radionational/programs/healthreport/ganfyd— the-sick-saga-of-sickness-certificates/3708930#transcript [Accessed 21 April 2018].

17. K. O'Brien, N. Cadbury, S. Rollnick and F. Wood (2008). 'Sickness certification in the general practice consultation: the patients' perspective, a qualitative study'. *Family Practice* 25:1 (20–6). Available at https://academic.oup.com/fampra/article/25/1/20/707693/Sickness-certification-in-the-general-practice [Accessed 19 November 2016].

18. NHS Digital (2017). 'Experimental Statistics: Fit Notes Issued by GP Practices, England. June 2017'. 27 October 2017. Available at https:// digital.nhs.uk/data-and-information/publications/statistical/fit-notes-issued-by-gp-practices/fit-notes-issued-by-gp-practices-england-june-2017 [Accessed 22 April 2018].

19. ONS (2017). 'Overview of the UK population: July 2017'. 21 July 2017. Available at https://www.ons.gov.uk/peoplepopulationandcommunity/populationandmigration/populationestimates/articles/overviewoftheukpopulation/july2017 [Accessed 22 April 2018].

20. Jaimie Kaffash (2016). 'Average waiting time for GP appointment increases 30% in a year'. *Pulse*, 10 June 2016. Available at http://www.pulsetoday.co.uk/your-practice/access/average-waiting-time-for-gp-appointment-increases-30-in-a-year/20032025.fullarticle [Accessed 19 November 2016].

21. J Archer et al. (2014). 'Understanding the rise in Fitness to Practise complaints from members of the public'. Report, Plymouth University Peninsula Schools of Medicine and Dentistry, 30 January 2014. Available online at http://www.gmc-uk.org/static/documents/content/Archer_et_al_FTP_Final_Report_30_01_2014.pdf [Accessed 6 August 2017]; GMC (2015). 'Fitness to Practice Statistics 2015'. Available at http://www.gmc-uk.org/DC9491_07___Fitness_to_Practise_Annual_Statistics_Report_2015___Published_Version.pdf_68148873.pdf [Accessed 6 August 2017].

22. GMC (2015). 'Fitness to Practice Statistics 2015'.

23. T. Bourne et al. (2015). 'The impact of complaints procedures on the welfare, health and clinical practise of 7926 doctors in the UK: a cross-sectional survey'. *BMJ Open.* Available at http://bmjopen.bmj.com/content/5/1/e006687 [Accessed 6 August 2017].

24. R.P.C. Handfield-Jones (1964). 'Who shall help the doctor? Ancillaries, prescriptions and certificates'. *Lancet* 2:1173.

10. THE LAND OF THE BLIND

1. Thomas Sydenham (1676). *Observationes mediciae morborum acutorum historiam et curiationem.* London: Kettilby. Available at https://archive.org/details/BIUSante_82971x01 [Accessed 4 May 2018].

2. K. Kroenke and A. D. Mangelsdorff (1989). 'Common Symptoms in Ambulatory Care: Incidence, Evaluation, Therapy and Outcome'. *American Journal of Medicine* 86 (262–6).

3. National Institutes of Health (2013). 'Factsheet: Human Genome Project'. 29 March 2013. Available at https://report.nih.gov/NIHfactsheets/ViewFactSheet.aspx?csid=45 [Accessed 2 September 2017].

4. Anon (1724). *Onania: or, the heinous sin of self-pollution and all its frightful consequences (in both sexes) considered with spiritual and physical advice to those who have already injured themselves by this abominable practice.* London: H. Cooke. The eighteenth edition of 1756 is available online at https://archive.org/details/b20442348 [Accessed 19 August 2017].

5. A. Comfort (1967). *The Anxiety Makers: Some Curious Preoccupations of the Medical Profession,* pp. 106–7. London: Thomas Nelson and Sons.

6. N. Burton (2015). 'When Homosexuality Stopped Being a Mental Disorder'. *Psychology Today,* 18 September 2015. Available at https://www.psychologytoday.com/blog/hide-and-seek/201509/when-homosexuality-stopped-being-mental-disorder [Accessed 19 August 2017].

7. S. Cartwright (1851). 'Diseases and Peculiarities of the Negro Race'. *De Bow's Review* XI. Reproduced and available on the Public Broadcasting Service website at http://www.pbs.org/wgbh/aia/part4/4h3106t.html [Accessed 19 August 2017].

8. B. Hunt (1855). 'Dr. Cartwright on "Drapetomania"'. *Buffalo Medical*

Journal 10 (438–42S). Available at https://books.google.co.uk/books ?id=coBYAAAAMAAJ&pg=PA438&redir_esc=y#v=onepage&q&f= false [Accessed 19 August 2017].

9. Public Health England (2016). 'Committee on Medical Aspects of Radiation in the Environment (COMARE): 17th Report'. Available at https://www.gov.uk/government/uploads/system/uploads/attachment_ data/file/554981/COMARE_17th_Report.pdf [Accessed 19 August 2017].

10. *The Telegraph* (2017). 'Council forced to pay £12k to man who lives in tent because he is "allergic" to electricity'. 6 July 2017. Available at http://www.telegraph.co.uk/news/2017/07/06/council-forced-pay-12k-man-lives-tent-allergic-electricity/ [Accessed 15 August 2017].

11. L McLaren (2000). 'Non-scents in Nova Scotia'. *The Globe and Mail*, 29 April 2000. Available at https://www.theglobeandmail.com/life/ non-scents-in-nova-scotia/article767434/ [Accessed 24 October 2018].

12. Cosmetics Design Europe (2008). 'US concern over fragrance use hits Europe'. 21 March 2008. Available at http://www.cosmeticsdesign-europe.com/Formulation-Science/US-concern-over-fragrance-use-hits-Europe [Accessed 15 August 2017]; Maggie O'Neill (2017). 'We're becoming ALLERGIC to the modern world: Thousands have been diagnosed with new mysterious condition that causes anxiety, sneezing and even seizures'. *Mail Online*, 25 October 2017. Available at https://www.dailymail.co.uk/health/article-5014369/The-illness-makes-women-allergic-modern-world.html [Accessed 5 November 2018].

13. World Health Organization (2018). 'International Statistical Classification of Diseases and Related Health Problems 11th Revision'. Available at https://icd.who.int/browse11/l-m/en [Accessed 23 June 2018]; American Psychiatric Association (2013). *Diagnostic and statistical manual of mental disorders* (5th ed.)

14. World Health Organization (2018). 'Gaming Disorder'. January 2018. Available at http://www.who.int/features/qa/gaming-disorder/en/ [Accessed 23 June 2018].

15. M. Moran (2013). 'Section III of New Manual Looks to Future'. *Psychiatric News*, 17 May 2013. Available at https://psychnews.psychi-

atryonline.org/doi/full/10.1176/appi.pn.2013.5b8 [Accessed 4 May 2018].

16. S. Viola and J. Moncrieff (2016). 'Claims for sickness and disability benefits owing to mental disorders in the UK: trends from 1995 to 2014'. *British Journal of Psychiatry Open* 2:1 (18–24). Available at https://www.cambridge.org/core/services/aop-cambridge-core/content/view/6DA7F0F56442BA881979BB81A6400D04/S2056472 400001101a.pdf/claims_for_sickness_and_disability_benefits_owing_to_mental_disorders_in_the_uk_trends_from_1995_to_2014.pdf [Accessed 24 October 2018].

17. Health and Safety Executive (2016). 'Work related Stress, Anxiety and Depression Statistics in Great Britain 2016'. Available at http://www.hse.gov.uk/statistics/causdis/stress/stress.pdf [Accessed 19 August 2017].

18. A. Newell and I. Gazeley (2012). 'The declines in infant mortality and fertility: Evidence from British cities in demographic transition'. Economics Department Working Paper Series No. 48–2012, University of Sussex. Available at https://www.sussex.ac.uk/webteam/gateway/file.php?name=wps-48–2012.pdf&site=24 [Accessed 12 September 2017]; ONS (2015). 'How has life expectancy changed over time?' 9 September 2015. Available at http://visual.ons.gov.uk/how-has-life-expectancy-changed-over-time/ [Accessed 12 September 2017].

19. BBC (undated). 'How do you fix a face that's been blown off by shrapnel?' Available at http://www.bbc.co.uk/guides/zxw42hv [Accessed 12 September 2017].

20. BBC (1969). 'Apollo 11: The Impact on Earth'. *Panorama*, first broadcast 21 July 1969. Available at https://www.bbc.co.uk/programmes/p0142pxj [Accessed 3 November 2018].

21. S. Ginn and J. Horder (2012). '"One in four" with a mental health problem: the anatomy of a statistic'. *BMJ Online*, 22 February 2012. Available at https://www.researchgate.net/profile/Stephen_Ginn/publication/221858556_One_in_four_with_a_mental_health_problem_The_anatomy_of_a_statistic/links/547de5900cf285ad5b08ae9a/One-in-four-with-a-mental-health-problem-The-anatomy-of-a-statistic.pdf [Accessed 15 September 2017].

22. Time to Change (2017). 'Myths/Facts'. Available at https://www.time-to-change.org.uk/mental-health-statistics-facts [Accessed 15 September 2017].

23. MIND (2017). 'Mental health facts and statistics'. April 2017. Available at https://www.mind.org.uk/information-support/types-of-mental-health-problems/statistics-and-facts-about-mental-health/how-common-are-mental-health-problems/#.WbwGwMbMzAx [Accessed 15 September 2017].

24. Parliament.uk (2017). 'House of Commons Library—Suicide: Summary of statistics'. 20 January 2017. Available at http://researchbriefings.parliament.uk/ResearchBriefing/Summary/CBP-7749 [Accessed 29 May 2018].

25. ONS (2017). 'Statistical bulletin—Suicides in the UK: 2016 registrations'. 18 December 2017. Available at https://www.ons.gov.uk/peoplepopulationandcommunity/birthsdeathsandmarriages/deaths/bulletins/suicidesintheunitedkingdom/2016registrations [Accessed 29 May 2018].

26. BBC News (2017). 'UK suicide rate shows largest drop for 20 years'. 18 December 2017. Available at http://www.bbc.co.uk/news/health-42393071 [Accessed 29 May 2018].

27. ONS (2017). 'Statistical bulletin—Suicides in the UK: 2016 registrations'.

28. Health and Social Care Act 2012, 64(3). Available at http://www.legislation.gov.uk/ukpga/2012/7/contents/enacted [Accessed 28 April 2018]; HMG (2015). 'NHS Constitution for England: resources'. Available at https://www.gov.uk/government/collections/nhs-constitution-for-england-resources [Accessed 28 April 2018]; HMG (2017). 'NHS mandate 2017 to 2018'. Available at https://www.gov.uk/government/publications/nhs-mandate-2017-to-2018 [Accessed 28 April 2018].

29. HMG (2017). 'Thriving at Work: The Stevenson/Farmer review of mental health and employers'. Available at https://www.gov.uk/government/uploads/system/uploads/attachment_data/file/654514/thriving-at-work-stevenson-farmer-review.pdf [Accessed 29 October 2017].

30. NHS Digital (2017). 'Prescriptions Dispensed in the Community'.

Available at https://files.digital.nhs.uk/publication/s/o/pres-disp-com-eng-2006-16-rep.pdf [Accessed 6 October 2018].

31. R. A. Charlton et al. (2014). 'Selective serotonin reuptake inhibitor prescribing before, during and after pregnancy: a population-based study in six European regions'. *British Journal of Obstetrics and Gynaecology*, 28 October 2014. Available at http://onlinelibrary.wiley.com/doi/10.1111/1471-0528.13143/epdf [Accessed 9 September 2017].

32. K. F. Huybrechts et al. (2013). 'National trends in antidepressant medication treatment among publicly-insured pregnant women'. *General Hospital Psychiatry* 35:3 (265–71). Available at https://www.ncbi.nlm.nih.gov/pmc/articles/PMC4077674/ [Accessed 9 September 2017].

33. NHS Digital (2017). 'Prescriptions Dispensed in the Community'.

34. D. Raj et al. (2017). 'Antidepressants during pregnancy and autism in offspring: population based cohort study'. *British Medical Journal* 358:8115. Available at http://www.bmj.com/content/bmj/358/bmj.j2811.full.pdf [Accessed 9 September 2017]; X. Liu et al. (2017). 'Antidepressant use during pregnancy and psychiatric disorders in offspring: Danish nationwide register based cohort study'. *British Medical Journal* 358:j3668. Available at http://www.bmj.com/content/bmj/358/bmj.j3668.full.pdf [Accessed 9 September 2017].

11. FANNING THE FLAMES

1. S. Hussey et al. (2003). 'Sickness certification system in the United Kingdom: qualitative study of views of general practitioners in Scotland'. *British Medical Journal*, 22 December 2003. Available at http://www.bmj.com/content/bmj/328/7431/88.full.pdf [Accessed 16 November 2016].

2. J. Owen (2006). 'Stephen Fry: The comic actor talks openly for the first time about the self-loathing brought about by his bipolar disorder'. *The Independent*, 17 September 2006. Available at https://www.independent.co.uk/life-style/health-and-families/health-news/stephen-fry-my-battle-with-mental-illness-416386.html [Accessed 26 October 2018].

3. D. Chan and L. Sireling (2010). '"I want to be bipolar" ... a new phenomenon'. *The Psychiatrist* 34 (103–5). Available at http://pb.rcpsych.org/content/34/3/103.short [Accessed 14 September 2017].

4. Andrew Malleson (2002). *Whiplash and other useful illnesses*, pp. 93–6. Montreal/Kingston: McGill-Queen's University Press; N. M. Hadler (1990). 'Cumulative trauma disorders. An iatrogenic concept'. *Journal of Occupational Medicine* 32 (38–41); M. Awerbuch (2004). 'Repetitive strain injuries: has the Australian epidemic burnt out?' *Internal Medicine Journal* 34:7 (416–19). Available at http://onlinelibrary.wiley.com/doi/10.1111/j.1444-0903.2004.00640.x/full [Accessed 14 September 2017].

5. Ministry of Justice (2017). 'Part 1 of the Government Response to: Reforming the Soft Tissue Injury ("Whiplash") Claims Process'. February 2017. Available at https://www.gov.uk/government/uploads/system/uploads/attachment_data/file/593431/part-1-response-to-reforming-soft-tissue-injury-claims.pdf [Accessed 15 September 2017].

6. G. Waddell and K. Burton (2001). 'Occupational health guidelines for the management of low back pain at work: evidence review'. *Occupational Medicine* 51:2 (124–35). Available at https://pdfs.semanticscholar.org/dff9/5228f2572c83fb7c1c3022e3e83ef38aef15.pdf [Accessed 20 August 2017].

7. Royal Mail (2017). 'Corporate Responsibility Report 2016/17'. Available at https://www.royalmailgroup.com/media/9769/royal-mail-group-plc-corporate-responsibility-report-2016-17.pdf [Accessed 26 October 2018].

8. Royal Mail (2016). 'Corporate Responsibility Report 2015/16'. Available at https://www.royalmailgroup.com/media/9770/royal-mail-group-plc-corporate-responsibility-report-2015-16.pdf [Accessed 26 October 2018].

9. The Mental Health Taskforce (2016). 'The five year forward view for mental health: a report from the independent Mental Health Taskforce to the NHS in England'. February 2016. Available at https://www.england.nhs.uk/wp-content/uploads/2016/02/Mental-Health-Taskforce-FYFV-final.pdf [Accessed 12 September 2017].

10. Department of Health (2016). 'New investment in mental health services'. 15 February 2016. Available at https://www.gov.uk/government/news/new-investment-in-mental-health-services [Accessed 11 September 2017].

11. A. Joseph (2017). 'But what would granny say?' Prince Harry criticises "older generation" for relying on the stiff upper lip and bottling up mental health problems'. *The Daily Mail*, 7 September 2017. Available at http://www.dailymail.co.uk/news/article-4863236/Prince-Harry-says-Britons-bottle-mental-health-problems.html [Accessed 11 September 2017].

12. NHS England (2016). 'NHS commits to major transformation of mental health care with help for a million more people'. 15 February 2016. Available at https://www.england.nhs.uk/2016/02/fyfv-mh/ [Accessed 11 September 2017].

13. NHS Digital (2017). 'Prescriptions Dispensed in the Community'. Available at https://files.digital.nhs.uk/publication/s/o/pres-disp-com-eng-2006-16-rep.pdf [Accessed 6 October 2018]; S. Viola and J. Moncrieff (2016). 'Claims for sickness and disability benefits owing to mental disorders in the UK: trends from 1995 to 2014'. *British Journal of Psychiatry Open* 2:1 (18–24). Available at https://www.cambridge.org/core/services/aop-cambridge-core/content/view/6DA7F0F56442 BA881979BB81A6400D04/S2056472400001101a.pdf/claims_for_sickness_and_disability_benefits_owing_to_mental_disorders_in_the_uk_trends_from_1995_to_2014.pdf [Accessed 24 October 2018]; Health and Safety Executive (2016). 'Work related Stress, Anxiety and Depression Statistics in Great Britain 2016'. Available at http://www.hse.gov.uk/statistics/causdis/stress/stress.pdf [Accessed 19 August 2017].

14. HMG (2016). 'Statement from the new Prime Minister Theresa May'. 13 July 2016. Available at https://www.gov.uk/government/speeches/statement-from-the-new-prime-minister-theresa-may [Accessed 11 September 2017].

15. R. Merrick (2017). 'Theresa May pledges an extra 10,000 staff for NHS mental health services, but with huge doubts over funding'. *The Independent*, 6 May 2017. Available at http://www.independent.co.uk/news/uk/politics/election-latest-mental-health-theresa-may-staff-10000-law-discrimination-depression-a7722046.html [Accessed 12 September 2017].

16. HMG (2017). 'PM: mental health training for teachers will "make a

real difference to children's lives'". 27 June 2017. Available at https://www.gov.uk/government/news/pm-mental-health-training-for-teachers-will-make-a-real-difference-to-childrens-lives [Accessed 12 September 2017].

17. HMG (2017). 'Young people to benefit from new mental health awareness course'. 18 August 2017. Available at https://www.gov.uk/government/news/young-people-to-benefit-from-new-mental-health-awareness-course [Accessed 12 September 2017].

18. S. Arie (2017). 'Simon Wessely: "Every time we have a mental health awareness week my spirits sink"'. *British Medical Journal* 358:j4305, 21 September 2017. Available at http://www.bmj.com/content/358/bmj.j4305 [Accessed 21 September 2017].

19. D. Campbell (2017). 'NHS "waving white flag" as it axes 18-week waiting time operation target'. *The Guardian*, 31 March 2017. Available at https://www.theguardian.com/society/2017/mar/31/nhs-surgery-target-operations-cancelled-simon-stevens [Accessed 12 September 2017].

20. F. Basaglia (2014). *La maggioranza deviante. L'ideologia del controllo sociale totale.* Milan: Baldini & Castoldi.

21. C. de Saussure (1902). *A foreign view of England in the reigns of George I and George II: The letters of Monsieur Cesar de Saussure to his family; translated and edited by Madame Van Muyden*, pp. 92–3. London: John Murray. Available at https://archive.org/details/foreignviewofeng00sausuoft [Accessed 10 September 2017].

22. The Stationery Office (2008). 'Working for a Healthier Tomorrow: Dame Carol Black's Review of the Health of Britain's Working Age Population'. Available at https://www.gov.uk/government/uploads/system/uploads/attachment_data/file/209782/hwwb-working-for-a-healthier-tomorrow.pdf [Accessed 5 November 2016].

23. The Stationery Office (2011). 'Health at Work: An Independent Review of Sickness Absence'. Available at https://www.gov.uk/government/uploads/system/uploads/attachment_data/file/181060/health-at-work.pdf [Accessed 5 November 2016].

12. DIAGNOSTIC INCONTINENCE

1. C. Schuster (1914). 'Report of the Departmental Committee on sick-

ness benefit claims under the National Insurance Act. Cd. 7687. National Health Insurance. London: HM Stationery Office. Available at https://archive.org/details/b21361125_001 [Accessed 4 May 2018].

2. NatCen Social Research (2013). 'British Social Attitudes 30'. Available at http://www.bsa.natcen.ac.uk/media/38723/bsa30_full_report_final.pdf [Accessed 6 November 2016].

3. T. Bourne et al. (2015). 'The impact of complaints procedures on the welfare, health and clinical practise of 7926 doctors in the UK: a cross-sectional survey'. *BMJ Open*. Available at http://bmjopen.bmj.com/content/5/1/e006687 [Accessed 6 August 2017].

4. V. Ward (2012). '"Some may think she has got away with it," says judge sentencing Margaret Moran over expenses'. *The Telegraph*, 14 December 2012. Available at http://www.telegraph.co.uk/news/newstopics/mps-expenses/9744621/Some-may-think-she-has-got-away-with-it-says-judge-sentencing-Margaret-Moran-over-expenses.html [Accessed 13 September 2017]; A (2011). 'MPs' expenses: Labour's Margaret Moran faces 21 charges'. *The Guardian*, 6 September 2011. Available at https://www.theguardian.com/politics/2011/sep/06/mps-expenses-margaret-moran-21-charges [Accessed 29 October 2018].

5. A. Pearson (2015). 'Forgive my cynicism at the timely onset of Lord Janner's "dementia"'. *The Telegraph*, 22 April 2015. Available at http://www.telegraph.co.uk/news/health/elder/11554636/Forgive-my-cynicism-at-the-timely-onset-of-Lord-Janners-dementia.html [Accessed 13 September 2017].

6. A (2017). 'AA boss fired over hotel punch-up blames booze and pills for "sustained attack"'. *The Telegraph*, 12 September 2017. Available at http://www.telegraph.co.uk/news/2017/09/12/aa-boss-fired-hotel-punch-up-blames-booze-pills-sustained-attack/ [Accessed 13 September 2017].

7. P. Cumberlidge (2015). 'Sh*t Life Syndrome is the problem we can't medicate'. *The Daily Mirror*, 7 August 2015. Available at http://www.mirror.co.uk/news/uk-news/shit-life-syndrome-nhs-doctor-6212214 [Accessed 5 November 2018].

8. A. Mikhailova (2018). 'Tory MP Johnny Mercer: My battles with mental illness—and how Army veterans are being exploited and failed'. *The

Telegraph, 7 May 2018. Available at https://www.telegraph.co.uk/politics/2018/05/06/military-charities-exploiting-soldiers-ptsd-says-tory-mp-johnny/ [Accessed 7 May 2018].

9. J. Kirkup (2015). 'Cynical about politicians? This speech by Johnny Mercer MP should make you think again'. *The Telegraph*, 2 June 2015. Available at https://www.telegraph.co.uk/news/politics/11646320/Cynical-about-politicians-This-speech-by-Johnny-Mercer-MP-should-make-you-think-again.html [Accessed 7 May 2018].

10. B. Ellery (2018). 'POUTRAGEOUS! Posing by the pool, sickness bug scammers who falsely claimed that they were poisoned by food at Spanish resort and have been hit with a £15k bill'. *The Daily Mail*, 17 March 2018. Available at http://www.dailymail.co.uk/news/article-5513789/Posing-pool-Benidorm-sickness-bug-scammers.html [Accessed 18 March 2018].

11. H. R. Eriksen et al. (1998). 'Prevalence of subjective health complaints in the Nordic European countries in 1993'. European Journal of Public Health 8:4 (294–8). Available at https://academic.oup.com/eurpub/article-lookup/doi/10.1093/eurpub/8.4.294 [Accessed 16 August 2017].

12. R.P.C. Handfield-Jones (1964). 'Who shall help the doctor? Ancillaries, prescriptions and certificates'. *Lancet* 2:1173.

13. Health and Safety Executive (2016). 'Work related Stress, Anxiety and Depression Statistics in Great Britain 2016'. Available at http://www.hse.gov.uk/statistics/causdis/stress/stress.pdf [Accessed 19 August 2017].

14. M. Seifert et al. (2016). 'How Workplace Fairness Affects Employee Commitment'. *MIT Sloan Management Review Magazine*, Winter 2016. Available at http://sloanreview.mit.edu/article/how-workplace-fairness-affects-employee-commitment/ [Accessed 10 September 2017].

15. HM Inspectorate of Constabulary (2016). 'HMIC Value for Money Profile 2016: Metropolitan Police Service'. Available at https://www.justiceinspectorates.gov.uk/hmicfrs/wp-content/uploads/metropolitan-2016-value-for-money-profile.pdf [Accessed 10 September 2017].

16. *Evening Standard* (2010). 'London boroughs where one in 10 police is off sick'. 18 August 2010. Available at https://www.standard.co.uk/news/london-boroughs-where-one-in-10-police-is-off-sick-6504330.html [Accessed 10 September 2017].

17. M. Wilkinson (2010). 'Too ill to go on the beat'. *The Oxford Times*, 26 February 2010. Available at http://www.oxfordtimes.co.uk/news/5032281.Too_ill_to_go_on_the_beat/ [Accessed 10 September 2017]; *Northampton Chronicle & Echo* (2009). 'One in 10 police officers "too sick" to work on the frontline'. 9 November 2009. Available at http://www.northamptonchron.co.uk/news/one-in-10-police-officers-too-sick-to-work-on-the-frontline-1–894945 [Accessed 10 September 2017].

18. A. Kirk (2014). 'Met police taking time off work with stress-related illnesses'. *The Guardian*, 28 December 2014. Available at https://www.theguardian.com/uk-news/2014/dec/28/met-police-time-off-work-stress-related-illnesses-days [Accessed 10 September 2017].

19. Home Office (2016). 'Police Workforce, England and Wales, 31 March 2016'. Statistical Bulletin 05/16, 21 July 2016. Available at https://www.gov.uk/government/uploads/system/uploads/attachment_data/file/544849/hosb0516-police-workforce.pdf [Accessed 10 September 2017].

20. Royal Mail (2017). 'Corporate Responsibility Report 2016/17'. Available at https://www.royalmailgroup.com/media/9769/royal-mail-group-plc-corporate-responsibility-report-2016–17.pdf [Accessed 26 October 2018].

21. I observed this in my time as a medical advisor to the police; anecdotal evidence can also be found at *The Sleeping Policeman* (2011). 'Complaints Against the Police'. *The Sleeping Policeman: A Former Police Officer's Blog*, 23 April 2011. Available at http://thethinkingpoliceman.blogspot.com/search/label/Complaints%20against%20police [Accessed 5 November 2018].

13. CONSENTING ADULTS

1. Health and Safety Executive (2016). 'Work related Stress, Anxiety and Depression Statistics in Great Britain 2016'. Available at http://www.hse.gov.uk/statistics/causdis/stress/stress.pdf [Accessed 19 August 2017].

2. E. Osborne (2013). *Reasonably Simple Economics: Why the World Works the Way It Does*, p. 298. New York: Apress.

3. D. Miller (2012). 'Think you've got a bad job? Indian "sewer diver" paid

just £3.50 a day (plus a bottle of booze) to unclog Delhi's drains'. *The Daily Mail*, 19 August 2012. Available at http://www.dailymail.co.uk/news/article-2190251/And-thought-bad-job-Indian-sewer-diver-paid-just-3–50-day-plus-bottle-booze-unclog-Delhis-drains.html [Accessed 16 September 2017].

4. J. Austin (2016). 'Back-breaking work for peanuts: why Brits won't slave on farms swamped by EU migrants'. *The Express*, 20 August 2016. Available at http://www.express.co.uk/news/uk/701860/Back-breaking-hell-paid-peanuts-why-Brits-won-t-slave-on-farms-swamped-by-EU-migrants [Accessed 16 September 2017].

5. ONS (2017). 'Statistical bulletin: UK labour market, September 2017'. Available at https://www.ons.gov.uk/employmentandlabourmarket/peopleinwork/employmentandemployeetypes/bulletins/uklabourmarket/latest [Accessed 15 September 2017].

6. C. Pratt (2018). 'The Law Explained: When is a Manager Responsible for Stress and Depression at Work?' Chartered Management Institute, 10 July 2018. Available at https://www.managers.org.uk/insights/news/2018/july/the-law-explained-when-is-a-manager-responsible-for-stress-and-depression-at-work [Accessed 5 November 2018].

14. STRESSFUL EXPERTS

1. G. Waddell, K. Burton, N. Kendall (2008). 'Vocational Rehabilitation: What works, for whom, and when?' University of Huddersfield, Evidence statement MH-12, p. 23. Available at http://eprints.hud.ac.uk/id/eprint/5575/1/waddellburtonkendall2008-VR.pdf [Accessed 26 September 2017].

2. S. Hussey et al. (2003). 'Sickness certification system in the United Kingdom: qualitative study of views of general practitioners in Scotland'. *British Medical Journal*, 22 December 2003. Available at http://www.bmj.com/content/bmj/328/7431/88.full.pdf [Accessed 16 November 2016]; J. Elms et al. (2005). 'The perceptions of occupational health in primary care'. *Occupational Medicine*, 1 September 2005. Available at https://academic.oup.com/occmed/article/55/7/523/1421931 [Accessed 16 November 2016].

3. Elms et al. (2005). 'The perceptions of occupational health in primary care'.

4. PwC (2012). 'Key trends in human capital 2012: A global perspective'. Available at https://www.pwc.com/gx/en/hr-management-services/pdf/pwc-key-trends-in-human-capital-management.pdf [Accessed 29 October 2017].

5. PwC (2014). 'A new vision for growth: Key trends in human capital 2014'. Available at https://www.pwc.com/gx/en/hr-management-services/pdf/pwc-key-trends-in-human-capital-2014.pdf [Accessed 29 October 2017].

6. HMG (2017). 'Thriving at Work: The Stevenson/Farmer review of mental health and employers'. Available at https://www.gov.uk/government/uploads/system/uploads/attachment_data/file/654514/thriving-at-work-stevenson-farmer-review.pdf [Accessed 29 October 2017].

7. HMG (2017). 'Police Remuneration Review Body report: 2017 England and Wales'. Available at https://www.gov.uk/government/publications/police-remuneration-review-body-report-2017 [Accessed 24 September 2017].

15. THE BLAME GAME

1. Australian Psychological Society (2016). 'Media release: Corporate psychopaths common and can wreak havoc in business, researcher says'. 13 September 2016. Available at https://www.psychology.org.au/news/media_releases/13September2016/Brooks/ [Accessed 27 September 2017]; P. Babiak, C. S. Neumann and R. D. Hare (2010). 'Corporate psychopathy: Talking the walk'. *Behavioral Sciences and the Law* 28:2 (174–93). Available at http://www.sakkyndig.com/psykologi/artvit/babiak2010.pdf [Accessed 27 September 2017].

16. SELF-HELP

1. H. Robertson (2015). 'The Health and Safety at Work Act turned 40'. *Occupational Medicine* 65 (176–9). Available at https://academic.oup.com/occmed/article/65/3/176/1481829 [Accessed 5 November 2018].

2. National Coal Mining Museum for England (2004). 'Statistics'. Available at https://ncm.org.uk/downloads/43/Statistics_In_Mining.pdf [Accessed 10 November 2016].

3. Hair and Beauty Industry Authority (2012). 'Industry Overview'.

Available at http://www.habia.org/industry/overview [Accessed 10 November 2016].

4. J. L. Weeks (1984). 'Export of Hazardous Industries: The View From a Local Union in the U.S.'. *Multinational Monitor* 5:9. Available at http://www.multinationalmonitor.org/hyper/issues/1984/09/weeks.html [Accessed 13 November 2016].

5. H. R. Eriksen et al. (1998). 'Prevalence of subjective health complaints in the Nordic European countries in 1993'. *European Journal of Public Health* 8:4 (294–8). Available at https://academic.oup.com/eurpub/article-lookup/doi/10.1093/eurpub/8.4.294 [Accessed 16 August 2017].

6. G. Waddell and A. K. Burton (2006). 'Is work good for your health and well-being?' London: The Stationery Office. Available at https://www.gov.uk/government/uploads/system/uploads/attachment_data/file/214326/hwwb-is-work-good-for-you.pdf [Accessed 31 July 2017]; G. Waddell, K. Burton, N. Kendall (2008). 'Vocational Rehabilitation: What works, for whom, and when?' University of Huddersfield, Evidence statement MH-12, p. 23. Available at http://eprints.hud.ac.uk/id/eprint/5575/1/waddellburtonkendall2008-VR.pdf [Accessed 26 September 2017].

7. K. Kroenke and A. D. Mangelsdorff (1989). 'Common Symptoms in Ambulatory Care: Incidence, Evaluation, Therapy and Outcome'. *American Journal of Medicine* 86 (262–6).

17. DEALING WITH REALITY

1. N. Hadler (May 1997). 'Back pain in the workplace: What you lift or how you lift matters far less than whether you lift or when'. *Spine* 22:9 (935–40).

2. Richard Johnstone (2018). 'Scottish Government civil servants could be next in line for "wellbeing hour"'. *Civil Service World*, 5 June 2018. Available at https://www.civilserviceworld.com/articles/news/scottish-government-civil-servants-could-be-next-line-'wellbeing-hour' [Accessed 8 June 2018].

18. LIMITS TO LAW

1. *Kapadia v. London Borough of Lambeth [1999]*. UKEAT 1004_98_2705

(27 May 1999). Available at http://www.bailii.org/uk/cases/UKEAT/ 1999/1004_98_2705.html [Accessed 30 April 2018].

2. Office for Disability Issues (2011). 'Equality Act 2010: Guidance on matters to be taken into account in determining questions relating to the definition of disability'. May 2011. Available at https://assets.publishing.service.gov.uk/government/uploads/system/uploads/attachment_data/file/570382/Equality_Act_2010-disability_definition.pdf [Accessed 31 October 2018].

3. Ibid.

4. Equality and Human Rights Commission (2011). 'Equality Act 2010: Employment Statutory Code of Practice'. January 2011. Available at http://intranet.yorksj.ac.uk/ucu/Equality%20documents/employercode.pdf [Accessed 31 October 2018].

5. This suggests that 'it would be sensible for employers not to attempt a fine judgment as to whether a particular individual falls within the statutory definition of disability'. Ibid.

6. N. Williams (2011). 'Assessing the damage: Assessing the Equality Act Impact Assessments'. Civitas, December 2011. Available at http://www.civitas.org.uk/content/files/equalityactimpact.pdf [Accessed 28 October 2017].

7. BBC News (2018). 'York teacher fired over film wins £646k payout'. 15 May 2018. Available at http://www.bbc.co.uk/news/uk-england-york-north-yorkshire-44130033 [Accessed 16 May 2018].

8. BDO United Kingdom (2017). 'UK productivity crisis deepens'. 9 April 2017. Available at https://www.bdo.co.uk/en-gb/news/2017/uk-productivity-crisis-deepens [Accessed 29 October 2017].

9. A. Allegretti (2017). 'Fury as Philip Hammond suggests disabled workers are suppressing economic productivity'. Sky News, 6 December 2017. Available at https://news.sky.com/story/fury-as-philip-hammond-suggests-disabled-workers-are-suppressing-economic-productivity-11159255 [Accessed 7 May 2018].

10. G. Heffer (2017). 'Charity's anger at PM's dismissal of Philip Hammond disability row'. Sky News. 13 December 2017. Available at https://news.sky.com/story/charitys-anger-at-pms-dismissal-of-philip-hammond-disability-row-11169200 [Accessed 7 May 2018].

11. Office for Disability Issues (2011). 'Equality Act 2010: Guidance on matters to be taken into account in determining questions relating to the definition of disability'.
12. Williams (2011). 'Assessing the damage'.
13. Department for Business, Energy & Industrial Strategy (2018). 'Business Population Estimates for the UK and Regions 2018'. 11 October 2018. Available at https://assets.publishing.service.gov.uk/government/uploads/system/uploads/attachment_data/file/746599/OFFICIAL_SENSITIVE_-_BPE_2018_-_statistical_release_FINAL_FINAL.pdf [Accessed 31 October 2018].
14. *Risby v. London Borough of Waltham Forest* UKEAT/0318/15/DM. Employment Appeal Tribunal ruling (18 March 2016). Available at https://www.employmentcasesupdate.co.uk/site.aspx?i=ed30986 [Accessed 31 October 2018].
15. J. Charlton (2016). 'Are "discrimination arising from disability" claims an easy route to employment tribunal wins?' *Personnel Today*, 5 October 2016. Available at https://www.personneltoday.com/hr/are-discrimination-arising-from-disability-claims-an-easy-route-to-employment-tribunal-wins/ [Accessed 10 June 2018].

19. THE NECESSARY MYTH

1. K. Kroenke and A. D. Mangelsdorff (1989). 'Common Symptoms in Ambulatory Care: Incidence, Evaluation, Therapy and Outcome'. *American Journal of Medicine* 86 (262–6).
2. J. Banks, R. Blundell and C. Emmerson (2015). 'IFS Working Paper W15/09. Disability benefit receipt and reform: reconciling trends in the United Kingdom'. Institute for Fiscal Studies, March 2015. Available at https://www.ifs.org.uk/uploads/publications/wps/WP201509.pdf [Accessed 19 November 2017].
3. J. R. Hampton et al. (1975). 'Relative contributions of history-taking, physical examination, and laboratory investigation to diagnosis and management of medical outpatients'. *British Medical Journal* 2 (486–9). Available at https://www.ncbi.nlm.nih.gov/pmc/articles/PMC1673456/pdf/brmedj01449-0038.pdf [Accessed 12 November 2017].
4. *ExaminerLive* (2006). 'Doctor suspended after "spying" claim'. 3

November 2006. Available at http://www.examiner.co.uk/news/west-yorkshire-news/doctor-suspended-after-spying-claim-5054180 [Accessed 12 November 2017].

20. THE LEAP OF FAITH

1. BBC News (2015). 'Glasgow bin lorry crash driver had "dizziness for decades"'. 31 July 2015. Available at http://www.bbc.co.uk/news/uk-scotland-glasgow-west-33732335 [Accessed 18 November 2016];). A. Sims (2016). 'Germanwings crash: Co-pilot Andreas Lubitz's final email reveals his "depression" and "fear of going blind"'. *The Independent*, 6 March 2016. Available at http://www.independent.co.uk/news/world/europe/germanwings-crash-co-pilot-andreas-lubitzs-final-email-reveals-depression-and-fear-of-going-blind-a6915736.html [Accessed 18 November 2016].

2. BBC News (2018). 'Coventry bus crash: Kailash Chander was driving dangerously'. 18 September 2018. Available at https://www.bbc.co.uk/news/uk-england-coventry-warwickshire-45561937 [Accessed 6 November 2018].

3. ONS (2018). 'Statistical bulletin: Employee earnings in the UK: 2018'. 25 October 2018. Available at https://www.ons.gov.uk/employmentandlabourmarket/peopleinwork/earningsandworkinghours/bulletins/annualsurveyofhoursandearnings/latest#analysis-of-employee-earnings [Accessed 1 November 2018].

4. Department for Work and Pensions (2013). 'Research Report No 841: Evaluation of the Statement of Fitness for Work (fit note): quantitative survey of fit notes'. June 2013. Available at https://www.gov.uk/government/uploads/system/uploads/attachment_data/file/273913/rrep841.pdf [Accessed 19 November 2017].

5. M. Hann and B. Sibbald (2013). 'Research Report No 835: General Practitioners' attitudes towards patients' health and work, 2010–12'. Department for Work and Pensions. Available at https://www.gov.uk/government/uploads/system/uploads/attachment_data/file/207514/rrep835.pdf [Accessed 19 November 2017].

6. DWP/Department of Health (2016). 'Improving Lives: The Work, Health and Disability Green Paper'. October 2016. Available at https://

www.gov.uk/government/uploads/system/uploads/attachment_data/file/564038/work-and-health-green-paper-improving-lives.pdf [Accessed 19 November 2017].

7. J. Elms et al. (2005). 'The perceptions of occupational health in primary care'. *Occupational Medicine*, 1 September 2005. Available at https://academic.oup.com/occmed/article/55/7/523/1421931 [Accessed 16 November 2016].

8. S. Lind (2016). 'Doctors call for patients to self-certify illness up to 14 days'. *Pulse*, 22 June 2016. Available at http://www.pulsetoday.co.uk/home/finance-and-practice-life-news/doctors-call-for-patients-to-self-certify-illness-up-to-14-days/20032139.fullarticle [Accessed 19 November 2017].

9. L. Donnelly (2016). 'Let workers sign themselves off sick for a fortnight say GPs, sparking fears of "skiver's charter"'. *The Telegraph*, 22 June 2016. Available at http://www.telegraph.co.uk/news/2016/06/22/let-workers-sign-themselves-off-sick-for-a-fortnight-say-gps-spa/ [Accessed 19 November 2017].

10. Ibid.; *HR News* (2016). 'BMA Calls for Longer Self-Certification Period Citing "Pressure Cooker" of GP Work'. 22 June 2016. Available at http://hrnews.co.uk/bma-calls-longer-self-certification-period-citing-pressure-cooker-gp-work/ [Accessed 19 November 2017].

11. The @Work Partnership (2017). 'Tea-breaker poll: sickness self-certification'. Press release, 7 December 2017. Available at https://www.atworkpartnership.co.uk/journal/press-releases/press-release-tea-breaker-poll-sickness-self-certification [Accessed 19 November 2017].

12. Faculty of Occupational Medicine/Society of Occupational Medicine (2017). 'Response to Improving Lives: The Work, Health and Disability Green Paper'. Joint Statement, 17 February 2017. Available at http://www.fom.ac.uk/wp-content/uploads/SOM-and-FOM-response-to-green-paper.pdf [Accessed 20 November 2017]; S. Lind (2016). 'Occupational health professionals reject GP calls to overhaul fit notes'. *Pulse*, 8 December 2016. Available at http://www.pulsetoday.co.uk/home/finance-and-practice-life-news/occupational-health-professionals-reject-gp-calls-to-overhaul-fit-notes/20033413.article [Accessed 19 November 2017].

13. Donnelly (2016). 'Let workers sign themselves off sick for a fortnight say GPs'; *HR News* (2016). 'BMA Calls for Longer Self-Certification Period Citing "Pressure Cooker" of GP Work'.

14. Shop, Distributive and Allied Employees' Association (undated). 'Info Sheet 12: Know your rights—sick leave'. Available at https://www.sda.com.au/media/12-KnowYourRights-SickLeave-PR.pdf [Accessed 21 April 2018].

15. F. Chung (2017). 'Calling in sick and getting away with it now costs only $20'. *mybody+soul*, 5 April 2017. Available at https://www.bodyandsoul.com.au/health/health-news/calling-in-sick-and-getting-away-with-it-now-costs-only-20/news-story/782580284e1dce5d3a6ffb4a40 3ec21b [Accessed 21 April 2018].

16. DWP/Department of Health (2017). 'Improving Lives: The Future of Work, Health and Disability'. White paper, November 2017. Available at https://assets.publishing.service.gov.uk/government/uploads/system/uploads/attachment_data/file/663399/improving-lives-the-future-of-work-health-and-disability.PDF [Accessed 7 November 2018].

17. T. Burchardt (1999). 'The Evolution of Disability Benefits in the UK: Re-weighting the basket'. Centre for Analysis of Social Exclusion, June 1999. Available at http://sticerd.lse.ac.uk/dps/case/cp/CASEpaper26.pdf [Accessed 1 December 2017].

18. National Audit Office (2016). 'Report by the Comptroller and Auditor General: Contracted-out health and disability assessments'. 8 January 2016. Available at https://www.nao.org.uk/wp-content/uploads/2016/01/Contracted-out-health-and-disability-assessments.pdf [Accessed 1 December 2017]. The DWP contracted the Centre for Health and Disability Assessments (CHDA), a wholly owned subsidiary of Maximus, to provide Work Capability Assessments for a 3.3-year period (2015–18), at a cost of £595 million. Actual expenditure was a little less, partly because CHDA struggled to meet the DWP's targets, and service credits were issued under the penalty terms within the contract.

19. D. Kraemer and H. Agerholm (2017). 'DWP spends £39m defending decisions to strip benefits from sick and disabled people'. *The Independent*, 28 August 2017. Available at http://www.independent.co.uk/news/uk/politics/dwp-disabled-people-benefits-legal-action-

lose-government-work-pensions-department-frank-field-mp-a7886166.html [Accessed 1 December 2017].
20. O. Wright (2013). 'Crackdown on disability benefits costs taxpayer £66m in appeals costs'. *The Independent*, 21 July 2013. Available at http://www.independent.co.uk/news/uk/politics/crackdown-on-disability-benefits-costs-taxpayer-66m-in-appeals-costs-8724779.html [Accessed 1 December 2018].
21. Work and Pensions Select Committee (2018). 'PIP and ESA Assessments', 12 February 2018. Available at https://publications.parliament.uk/pa/cm201719/cmselect/cmworpen/829/82909.htm [Accessed 4 November 2018].

21. A SORT OF LIFE

1. J. D'Onfro (2016). 'Jeff Bezos thinks that to save the planet we'll need to move all heavy industry to space'. *Business Insider*, 1 June 2016. Available at http://uk.businessinsider.com/jeff-bezos-on-blue-origin-and-space-2016-6 [Accessed 1 December 2017].
2. The Marmot Review (2010). 'Fair Society, Healthy Lives'. February 2010. http://www.parliament.uk/documents/fair-society-healthy-lives-full-report.pdf [Accessed 7 November 2018].
3. R. E. Cytowic (2017). 'There is a new link between screen-time and autism'. *Psychology Today*, 29 June 2017. Available at https://www.psychologytoday.com/gb/blog/the-fallible-mind/201706/there-is-new-link-between-screen-time-and-autism [Accessed 7 October 2018].
4. W. Beveridge (1906). 'The Problem of the Unemployed'. *The Sociological Review* 3:1 (323–41). Available at http://journals.sagepub.com/doi/pdf/10.1177/0038026106SP300130 [Accessed 3 May 2018].
5. Erika Lucas (2017). 'Unlimited annual leave: PR exercise or game changer?' Cezanne, 2 March 2017. Available at https://cezannehr.com/hr-blog/2017/03/unlimited-annual-leave-pr-exercise-or-game-changer/ [Accessed 19 November 2017].
6. LinkedIn (2017). 'LinkedIn Top Companies 2017: Where the world wants to work now'. 18 May 2017. Available at https://www.linkedin.com/pulse/linkedin-top-companies-2017-where-us-wants-work-now-daniel-roth [Accessed 19 November 2017].

INDEX

Aberhart, William, 161, 162, 291
Afghanistan War (2001–14), 146
Aldiss, Brian, 118–19
Alexander, Daniel 'Danny', 161
angor animi, 206
antidepressants, 124–5, 128, 234
Apollo XI moon landing (1969),
    118
Arbeit macht frei, 28
artificial intelligence (AI), 162,
    291
As Good as It Gets, 230
Attlee, Clement, 32, 61–2, 74, 81
automation, 12, 162, 202, 222,
    283, 291–5
Automobile Association, 143

back pain, 148, 169, 203–4, 211,
    222, 259
Bader, Douglas, 27, 34–5, 54
Basaglia, Franco, 138–9
Bashford, Henry, 84–5
Berne, Eric, 168

Bevan, Aneurin, 57, 59, 74–5,
    77, 80
Beveridge Report, 31–3
Beveridge, William, 34, 56, 58,
    63, 294
    benefit dependency, fears of, 33
    on children of unemployed,
        58, 294
    perceptions of, 34, 58
Bevin, Ernest, 58
Bezos, Jeff, 283–4
biopsychosocial model, 18, 209
Black, Carol, 35–9, 55, 81, 139
Black-Frost report, 139
Blair, Anthony 'Tony', 66–7
Blake, William, 61, 210
blue flu, 90
Bornstein, Harold, 90
Borsi, Giosué, 48
Brent, David, 216
British Disease, The, 254
British Medical Association,
    58–60, 275

337

INDEX

British Motor Museum, 290
British Social Attitudes survey, 5
Brown, Gordon, 95
Burton, Kim, 177, 209
Butler, Nicholas, 176

Caffeine Use Disorder, 111
Cameron, David, 37, 136
capitalism, 162
Cartwright, Samuel, 108–9
certification
    absurd examples of, 46–8
    as a cause of sickness, 266
    conflict of interest, 55, 262
    conflicting expectations for
        doctors, 74
    and exploitation, 267
    history of, 46, 49–52
    lawyers and, 256, 260
    as legitimisation of inactivity,
        253
    literary depiction of, 75–6, 79
    patient's judgement and, 94,
        100, 259
    politicians and, 260
    primary care, drain on, 92,
        95–6, 258, 266, 275
    projection and, 94
    safety-critical environment and,
        198–9, 267–70
    self-certification, 90, 275, 276
    sickness versus disease, 87
    statistics, 96
    straw-men arguments, 276
    trade unions and, 54, 256

and training, lack of, 94, 274
trust in doctors and, 49–52,
    131, 262
Chartered Institute of Personnel
    and Development, 69
Chartered Management Institute,
    170
Chronic Fatigue Syndrome
    (CFS), 82, 105
Churchill, Winston, 62
Citadel, The (Cronin), 74–7, 79,
    82, 257, 260, 275
Citizens Advice, 267
Civitas, 240, 242
Confederation of British Industry
    (CBI), 5, 69, 70, 277
Corporate Manslaughter and
    Corporate Homicide Act
    (2007), 202
Cooling, Nicholas, 260–61
Corbyn, Jeremy, 162
covert surveillance, 8, 29, 56, 261
Cox, Brian, 284
Cronin, Archibald, 74–8, 80
    Citadel, The, 74–7, 79, 82, 257,
        260, 275

Darwin, Charles, 116
Dawkins, Richard, 116, 117
Delvaux, Mady, 162
Department for Work and
    Pensions, 6, 13
    anonymising effect of, 13
    data, 6
    Health, Work and Wellbeing,
        139

INDEX

Ministry of National Insurance, forerunner of, 13

suicides of benefit applicants, 39

Work Capability Assessments, 39

depression, 120, 126, 133, 135, 136, 142–3, 207, 230

antidepressants, 124–5, 128, 234

diabetic diet analogy (for managing ill employees), 214–15

Diagnostic and Statistical Manual of Mental Disorders (DSM-V), 110–12, 120

disability benefits, 21, 28, 66, 279–81

doctors

as priests, 51–2

complaints about, 77, 79, 97–8, 144

lack of training in assessing sickness, 94

perceptions of certification, 92, 99–100, 275–8

perceptions of NHS, 93

time pressures upon, 95

trust in, 51, 78, 132, 142, 262

Does He Take Sugar? (paradigm), 219–21

drapetomania, 108, 132, 183, 254

Economic Man, 4, 23, 73

economy, 161

automation, 12, 162, 202, 222, 283, 291–5

as a driver of sickness, 5, 65, 67, 69, 83, 86

changing nature of, 86, 115, 162, 181–2, 201, 222, 284–6, 289–95

manufacturing, 114, 204, 289–90

service economy, 69, 115, 198, 267, 286, 290

small or medium sized enterprises (SMEs), 243, 245

electromagnetic hypersensitivity syndrome, 109

Elizabethan Poor Laws, 12, 279

Employee Assistance Programmes (EAPs), 175, 178

employees

management attempts to discredit, 221

manager engagement, 152, 164, 194, 211, 214, 221, 254, 271, 285, 289

suicide threats, 188–9, 195

Employment and Support Allowance (ESA), 16, 26, 29

Courts and Tribunals Service, cost to, 282

Regulation 35(2)(b), 39, 40

and Work Capability Assessment, 40, 68

employment tribunals, 229–49

Equality Act (2010), 154, 230–49

direct discrimination, 246

positive discrimination, 230–31, 238, 243

339

INDEX

INDEX

INDEX

INDEX

INDEX